Physical Assessment of Patients
The Byron Physical Assessment Framework

Physical Assessment of Patients

The Byron Physical Assessment Framework

Ruth Harris

Research Fellow, Florence Nightingale School of Nursing and Midwifery, King's College, London

Consulting Editor

Brian Dolan

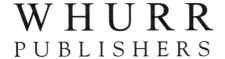

WHURR
PUBLISHERS

© 2002 Whurr Publishers Ltd
First published 2002 by
Whurr Publishers Ltd
19b Compton Terrace, London N1 2UN,
England, and 325 Chestnut Street, Philadelphia,
PA 19106, USA

British Library Cataloguing in Publication Data
A catalogue record for this book is available from the British Library.

ISBN 1 86156 288 8

Printed and bound in the UK by Athenaeum Press ltd, Gateshead, Tyne & Wear

Contents

Foreword   vii
Acknowledgements   ix
Preface   xi
Introduction   xv

CHAPTER 1   1

Assessment tools

CHAPTER 2   19

Development and refinement of the Byron Physical
Assessment Framework

CHAPTER 3   39

Evaluation of the reliability of the Byron Physical
Assessment Framework

CHAPTER 4   65

Evaluation of the validity of the Byron Physical Assessment
Framework

CHAPTER 5   73

Discussion

Appendix 1   87

Physical assessment teaching information for staff

Appendix 2   91

Second version of the NLIU Physical Assessment Framework

Appendix 3   93

First version of the NLIU Physical Assessment Framework

Appendix 4   95

Abnormal physiological signs and symptoms of the
cardiovascular system

Appendix 5   99

Abnormal physiological signs and symptoms of the neurological
system

Appendix 6   103

Abnormal physiological signs and symptoms of the
gastrointestinal system

Appendix 7   107

Abnormal physiological signs and symptoms of the
genitourinary system

Appendix 8   111

Definition of items on the Byron Physical Assessment
Framework before refinement by expert group

Appendix 9   117

Definition of items on the Byron Physical Assessment
Framework after refinement by expert group

References   137
Index   145

Foreword

This book should be useful for all those attempting to construct and validate clinical assessment and measuring tools. Ruth Harris has the expertise necessary to do this in a sophisticated yet realistic way for practice colleagues. This assessment tool, used on a nurse-led unit, was fundamental to safe and effective practice, giving evidence that the assessment process itself provides essential information that influences the quality of care provided. It provides an excellent model of practice-based research for the benefit of patients.

Professor Jenifer Wilson-Barnett
Head of School
Florence Nightingale School of Nursing and Midwifery
King's College, London

Acknowledgements

I would like to thank the following people:

- Professor Jenifer Wilson-Barnett and Peter Griffiths for their advice and support in supervising the study
- Peter Milligan for advice and guidance with the statistical analysis
- South East Thames Regional Health Authority who provided funding for the MSc course
- all the patients who agreed to participate in the study
- all the nursing staff who participated in the study
- the team on the nursing development unit (NDU), particularly Jonathan Williams, Sadie Collison, Ben Lewis, Karen Spilsbury and Fiona Miller
- and finally, Lyn Batehup and Amanda Evans, whose leadership of the NDU gave us all opportunities critically to appraise and develop our practice both individually and as a team.

Preface

The main aim of this study was to evaluate the reliability and validity of the Byron Physical Assessment Framework (BPAF) developed by a nursing development unit (NDU) to guide nurses in systematically assessing patients. As the BPAF had already been in use for over two years, a non-experimental, evaluative approach was taken.

Overall, the aims were to:

- examine the content and conceptual basis of the BPAF and make any necessary changes to refine it
- test the reliability of the BPAF by examining agreement between assessors
- teach a novice to use the BPAF and examine inter-rater reliability between the novice and an experienced assessor
- examine patient assessment documentation retrospectively for evidence of action taken as a result of using the BPAF as an indication of its validity.

The study was divided into three phases. The initial phase dealt with the first aim of the study and involved scrutinizing the BPAF to describe its purpose, conceptual basis and how it was developed. The BPAF was then refined using extensive literature review and expert opinion to improve its comprehensiveness and clarity for its intended purpose. As a result, the content validity of the BPAF was supported.

Phase two dealt with the second and third aims of the study, and involved a statistical analysis of inter-rater agreement, computing % agreement and Cohen's Kappa correlation for nominal data and standard deviation, 95% tolerance interval for the difference between assessors' scores and 95% confidence interval for the mean of these differences. The differences in scores of assessments conducted by a novice and an experienced assessor were compared to those of two experienced assessors. The inter-rater reliability of the nominal data items of the BPAF was found to be generally good, although the inter-rater reliability of the ratio items was disappointing. With relatively little teaching, novice assessors were able to use the BPAF and achieve good inter-rater reliability with experienced assessors, although this was lower than the reliability between two experienced assessors.

Phase three dealt with the fourth aim. As an indication of validity, the utilization of the BPAF in relation to its intended purpose was assessed by examining completed assessments and the outcome in terms of nurses' actions in light of new abnormal findings. The rate of completion and evidence of action taken by nurses was fair, showing that the BPAF does affect the actions of nurses, although it could be utilized more.

The study identified that the BPAF has potential as a physical assessment tool, although the method of assessing items with lower inter-rater reliability needs to be closely examined to reduce this variability. In addition, the reasons for both non-completion of the tool and lack of subsequent action on abnormal findings need to be addressed.

Phase of study / objectives	Conceptual analysis	Statistical analysis
Phase one 1 To review and describe the initial development, conceptual basis and purpose of the BPAF 2 To examine the content of the BPAF and revise as necessary to improve its comprehensiveness and clarity for its intended purpose	• literature review • expert opinion	—
Phase two 1 To examine inter-rater reliability between two independent assessors using the BPAF to assess assess patients being cared for on the NLIU 2 To assess whether this inter-rater reliability is stable over time 3 To examine inter-rater reliability between expert assessors while assessing patients on acute wards 4 To teach two novice assessors how to use the BPAF 5 To assess inter-rater reliability between one expert and one novice assessor 6 To assess reliability as a whole incorporating all the assessments carried out	—	*Nominal data* • Cohen's Kappa • % agreement *ratio data* • standard deviation • 95% confidence interval for the mean of the differences between assessors' scores • 95% tolerance interval for the difference between assessors' scores
Phase three 1 To examine the process used to refine the BPAF to establish whether content validity is supported 2 To retrospectively examine completed BPAFs to assess how consistently they are completed 3 To retrospectively examine patient documentation for evidence of action taken by nurses as a result of the detection of a new abnormality using the BPAF to assess utilization of the BPAF	• literature review • expert opinion	• descriptive statistics (%)

Introduction

Patient assessment can be seen as a prerequisite for the provision of individualized and appropriate nursing care. Kratz (1979) describes assessment as a deliberate, systematic collection of information about a patient, based on predetermined topics. Numerous assessment tools or frameworks have been developed to enhance nurses' assessment. They guide the collection of information about the patient and, in some cases, help nurses make decisions about the nursing care patients need. However, the reliability and validity of many of the tools designed for use in clinical settings are highly questionable and this must cast doubt on their value and, moreover, whether they should be relied upon to guide clinical decisions affecting patient care (Mallick 1981).

In February 1993, a nursing development unit (NDU) established a nursing-led service for medical inpatients (the nursing-led inpatient unit, NLIU), whereby medically stable patients with significant nursing needs are transferred to the care of a primary nurse who takes responsibility for co-ordinating the remainder of the patient's hospital stay (Evans and Griffiths 1994). However, 'medical stability' was recognized to be a transient phenomenon and it was therefore deemed essential for nursing staff to systematically review their patients each day to detect any changes in their physical condition and arrange timely medical input during one of the unit doctor's sessions. To facilitate this, the nursing staff developed a physical assessment framework, the Byron Physical Assessment Framework (BPAF). This framework takes a systems approach, and while it was thought to be inappropriate for nurses to diagnose, it should help them to identify and articulate deviations from the patient's norm and make appropriate referrals based on this information.

An interim report of a randomized controlled study to evaluate the effectiveness of the nurse-led service has shown that patients cared for on the NLIU were less physically dependent at discharge, less likely to develop a pressure sore and less likely to develop a chest or urinary tract infection than a comparative group of patients cared for in the traditional way on acute wards (Griffiths and Evans 1995). Although no possible reasons for the improved outcomes have been discussed, anecdotal suggestions from the nurses on the NLIU include the regular, comprehensive assessment facilitated by the BPAF.

The assessment framework has a second purpose, which is to aid screening of suitable patients prior to transfer to the nursing-led unit. Obviously, if a patient has ongoing medical needs it would be unwise for the NLIU to accept responsibility for that patient's care until these needs have been met. Therefore it can be seen that the physical assessment framework serves two purposes, both of which help the nursing staff make decisions about how best to fulfil patient need. However, in line with Mallick's (1981) criticism of clinical assessment tools, there has been no testing of this assessment framework for reliability and validity. In light of this, the testing of the NLIU BPAF would appear to be of utmost importance, especially as it has been in clinical use for over two years.

This study tests the BPAF for reliability and validity. As the use of the BPAF was already well established in the clinical area, an evaluative, non-experimental approach was taken. The study had the following aims:

1 To examine the content and conceptual basis for the assessment framework and make any necessary changes to refine it.
2 To test the reliability of the BPAF by examining agreement between assessors.
3 To teach a novice to use the BPAF and examine inter-rater reliability between the novice and an experienced assessor.
4 To examine patient assessment documentation retrospectively for evidence of action taken as a result of using the BPAF as an indication of the BPAF's validity.

Chapter 1
Assessment tools

Intr

become a very familiar concept in nursing. y new term for the profession, the importance of its t. been recognized. Florence Nightingale and many inf ce have stressed the importance of accurate observat to the extent that 'If you cannot get the habit of or other, you had better give up being a nurse, ng, however kind and anxious you may be' (Nigh despite being a 'household' concept in nursing, the theoretical underpinning of assess-ment is ...ced. Reed (1989) suggests that the process of nursing ...sment has not been fully explored and Pank (1994) describes the understanding of nursing assessment as 'tenuous'.

The purpose of this chapter is to give a brief definition of nursing assessment and explore some of the difficulties experienced by practising nurses in the area of assessment. The main focus of the chapter, however, is the development and testing of assessment tools and frameworks in nursing.

Theoretical description of assessment

The idea that nursing care should be based on the careful assessment of the patient's condition was brought to prominence when care planning based on 'the nursing process' was introduced into the UK during the 1970s. The idea that care should aim to meet the identified needs of individual patients was readily accepted by nurses, partly because of their dissatisfaction with depersonalized, task-oriented care (de la Cuesta 1983) and partly because they saw it as a way of attaining professional status for nursing.

Tierney (1984) has described assessment, the first stage of the nursing process, as comprising of the three following activities:

1

- collecting information (data)
- reviewing the data collected
- and identifying the patient's problems from the data.

McFarlane and Castledine (1982) refer to data collection as separate from assessment. Similarly Marks-Maran (1983) divides assessment into two steps: data collection and nursing diagnosis. The Nursing Process Evaluation Working Group (NPEWG 1986) refers to assessment as involving the gathering of information about a patient from a variety of sources by a variety of means. Hurst et al. (1991) differentiate between problem identification, which is the initial gathering and analysing of data leading to the identification of problems, and assessment, which is a deeper, problem-specific, systematic collection of data enabling a greater understanding of the problem, its magnitude and how it relates to other problems.

Assessment is arguably the most important stage of nursing. It forms the basis for any planned nursing intervention (Barker 1987) and a baseline against which subsequent events in the hospital stay can be compared (Tierney 1984). Tierney also considers assessment to be vital to the development of the nurse-patient relationship. Establishing a rapport between the nurses and patient sets the groundwork for 'partnership in care' and thus improves the quality of the assessment data. Although assessment is described as a step in the nursing process or referred to as 'an assessment' or 'the assessment procedure', this is misleading, because assessment should never be a once-only event (Tierney 1984). In reality, assessment is an ongoing activity whereby the patient is continually reviewed and care reappraised to ensure that patient's needs are being met.

The reality of assessment in practice

Walsh (1991) considered that patient assessment was often poorly carried out. It was frequently seen as synonymous with admission, to the extent that many nurses talked of admitting rather than assessing a new patient. As a result, the occurrence of ongoing assessment, which is vital to monitor the success of care and detect the emergence of new problems, was unlikely. Likewise NPEWG (1986) found evidence that suggested that assessment was conducted in a routine manner with little thought of purpose. They found that patient assessment was seen as a form-filling exercise, which resulted in the unnecessary duplication of questions and the collection of inappropriate information that was not used. They also found that reassessment after initial admission assessment was rarely achieved. This over-reliance on routine and ritualistic thinking in patient assessment has also been identified by Walsh and Ford (1989), in the area of 'doing the obs'. They questioned why apyrexial patients often had their temperature taken up to six times a day or why patients so frequently had a constant improbably rapid respiratory rate of 20 breaths/minute. This, they proposed, suggested that nursing assessment was less than expert, and did not take patients' needs into consideration.

As a result of the nursing assessment being regarded as a reference sheet containing patient information rather than the foundation for a nursing problem statement and an individualized care plan, de la Cuesta (1983) found that care plans tended to focus largely on physical care based on medical diagnosis. She attributed this to the failure of nurses to accept the ideological changes that emphasize meeting patients' individual, comprehensive needs in a flexible, dynamic way, and which are inherent in the nursing process.

In a similar way, Reed and Bond (1991) found that assessment and care planning was restricted by an inappropriate 'medical' model of care. In their study, they found that in long-term care of the elderly wards, nurses still evaluated their work by the yardstick of cure. In these wards where cure was unlikely, the nurses did not value what they did and as a result sought satisfaction primarily from giving 'good geriatric care', which was achievable but involved speedy and efficient completion of ward routines, precluding the assessment of individual patients' problems.

The need for a model of care

These difficulties experienced by practising nurses may reflect a misunderstanding of the purpose of the nursing process. It is not a model of nursing, but has been described by Aggleton and Chalmers (1986) as 'a set of systematic steps that can be gone through in planning and delivering care'. Likewise, Pearson and Vaughan (1986) describe the nursing process as a 'vehicle' through which nursing is delivered, and maintain that this process does not infer any definition or content as to what the package of nursing involves. A model of nursing is essential to give guidance concerning what to assess, how to plan and implement care, and how to evaluate the care given. Without such explicit statements of belief there can be little understanding of what assessment information is required (Coles and Fullenwider 1988). Riehl and Roy (1980) have defined a nursing model as 'a systematically constructed, scientifically based, and logically related set of concepts which identify components of nursing practice, together with the theoretical basis of the concepts and values required for their use by the practitioner'. Similarly

Pearson and Vaughan (1986) describe a nursing model as being 'made up of the components or ideas which go towards making up nursing – what it is, the beliefs, the values and the theories and concepts on which it is built'.

Many models for nursing practice have been developed: Henderson (1966), Roy (1980), Roper et al. (1980), Rogers (1970) and Orem (1991) to name but a few. However, all these models have been heavily criticized. They are seen as unrealistic, representing the views of a minority of academic nurses as to what nursing ought to be (Wright 1990). Some models are seen as reductionist and dehumanizing (Walsh 1990), others as jargonistic and pretentious (Wright 1990). But regardless of whether a practice area uses an existing published model of nursing, each team member will have his or her own ideas of what nursing actually is, what the role of the nurse is and, as a consequence, the type of care that should be given to patients. Pearson and Vaughan (1986) argue that it is paramount that these ideas are discussed and agreement reached as to what constitutes nursing and is the most appropriate way to give nursing care for each particular area or client group. As a result, they purport that the continuity of care patterns and treatment will increase by giving direction to nursing care, since the goals of nursing work will be understood by the whole team. Moreover, Wright (1986) stresses the importance that models should be seen to help nurses explore and define their work and should not confine them to a set order.

Returning to the long-term care wards in Reed and Bond's (1991) study, it can be seen that acceptance of an inappropriate model of care can be instrumental in restricting individual patient assessment and the provision of therapeutic nursing care. The conflict of a 'cure' philosophy in an area where cure is unlikely can have a damaging effect on nurse morale and feelings of professional worth. As one nurse said, '... we're all dressed up with nowhere to go. Here we are in hospital, all the gear, all the equipment, all in uniform, all the rules and regulations but we don't do what a hospital does... we look like a hospital, but we don't get anybody better so we're not'. In contrast, Faucett et al. (1990) investigated the effect of using Orem's self-care model on nursing care in a nursing home setting. While further study was recommended, preliminary findings suggest that nursing staff using Orem's model differ in their nursing assessments and goals of care, tending to be more specific and reflect more resident participation in care.

Therefore a model of care can be damaging or empowering, depending on the way it is used. Adopted in an unthinking, inflexible, 'all or nothing' way, a model is unlikely to affect the practice of nursing and will become just another ritual (Ford and Walsh 1994).

Use of structured assessment tools

In a similar way to how nursing models give structure to patient assessment and the provision of nursing care, assessment tools can be seen as giving structure to assessment and thus reinforcing the model on which they are based (Lewis 1988). Mulhearn (1989) found that unstructured nursing assessments were haphazard and dependent on nurses' knowledge, experience, sense of personal organization and daily work pressure, while a structured assessment format assisted the collection of comprehensive information about patients as individuals. Similarly, Batehup and Evans (1992) found little documented evidence of continuing assessment, with the exception of problems where structured assessment formats, e.g. wound and pain management protocols, were used. This suggests that a structured assessment tool aids the assessment process itself and/or the documentation of assessment, either of which would ultimately improve patient care. Tanner (1982) suggests that when nurses are told what to look for, they will make more appropriate observations and interpret them more accurately.

Assessment tools will only improve assessment if they are accurate and comprehensive. Since clinical decisions will be made on the basis of the assessment, it is of crucial importance that they are carefully developed and tested. This emphasizes the importance of testing in full the nursing-led inpatient unit (NLIU) physical assessment framework (the Byron Physical Assessment Framework, BPAF) that has been in clinical use for over two years.

Main literature search

A literature search was conducted to explore the area of literature concerning physical assessment frameworks. The sources of the search included CINHAL 1/82-10/94 International Research Index, Medline and the Royal College Nursing Database. Some search headings, such as 'patient assessment', yielded too many articles. Therefore combinations of headings, such as 'nursing diagnosis', 'patient assessment', 'instrument construction', 'clinical assessment tool', were searched. Peer-reviewed or core nursing journals were selected so that research studies would be identified.

The search did not find any physical assessment tools similar to the BPAF. This was interesting, and is possibly due to the perceived 'medical function' of physical assessment and the movement of interest to areas where nursing can function independently. Medical literature tended to focus on diagnostic treatment protocols rather than clinical examination protocols. However, tools that assessed different aspects of a patient's condition were found. It was decided to review these studies to explore the area of development and testing of physical assessment tools. Functional assessment tools were not reviewed as they are more concerned with patients' physical ability than their physical condition. Similarly pressure sore risk assessment scales were not reviewed.

Of the several hundred studies identified, 34 were selected on the grounds that they appeared to be concerned with the development and testing of physical assessment tools. On closer examination, 12 reports were discarded as less relevant, e.g. literature reviews, reports of screening programmes, reports of documentation audits. Severity of illness measurement scales were also discarded, as the rationale for their development was concerned with the management of resources rather than patient assessment per se.

This review of the development and testing of the 22 assessment tools selected will take the format used by McDowell and Newell (1987) in their extensive review of functional assessment scales, discussing the studies collectively with regard to purpose, conceptual basis, how developed, reliability and validity. It is not possible to describe all the studies in detail, but various aspects will be discussed to illustrate points made about tool development.

The purpose of assessment tools

The purpose of an assessment tool is concerned with what the tool was designed to do and the types of person it is intended for, specifying age and diagnostic group. The more specific the purpose, the easier it is to judge whether the tool has achieved its aim. The purpose of most of the assessment tools reviewed was to improve the quality and accuracy of the assessment made, and the impetus for the development of the tool was the perceived inadequacy of existing assessments. For example, the Western Consortium for Cancer Nursing Research (WCCNR 1991) developed a staging system for the assessment of chemotherapy-induced stomatitis to clarify the different stages and to encourage clinicians to make more holistic assessments. Similarly, Miller (1990) introduced the incontinence monitoring record, which provided nursing assistants with an easier and more comprehensive method of recording incontinence patterns.

Several of the assessment tools reviewed aimed to facilitate identification of abnormal symptoms, which would enable timely intervention and therefore prevent acute crisis. For example, the Moller-Murphy Symptom Management Assessment Tool (Murphy and Moller 1993) was designed to identify and communicate the frequency, intensity and duration of psychiatric symptoms that indicate relapse, in order to initiate a change in management to prevent the symptoms from becoming severe enough to disrupt daily activities. And Crandall and Getchell-Reiter (1993) developed a guide to assess early signs of sepsis in neonates.

The prediction of risk was another reason for the development of some tools. Brians et al. (1991) developed a tool to predict the discharge needs of patients over 65 years. Although not specified by any of the studies reviewed, it can be seen that the use of good assessment tools can collate comprehensive, pertinent assessment data and enable health professionals to make decisions about the treatment and management of patients' health needs.

The majority of the assessment tools reviewed measured just one construct, for instance feeding problems in patients with dementia (Watson 1994), constipation (McMillan and Williams 1989), urinary symptoms (Petrucci et al. 1992). Only four of the tools aimed to assess multiple constructs. Three of these were designed to assess patients' nursing needs according to specific models of care, e.g. Rogers (1970) Science of Unitary Beings (Tettero et al. 1993). The fourth study, Chang et al. (1988), developed a general assessment guide for identifying nursing diagnoses based on the North American Nursing Diagnosis Associations Taxonomy I.

Conceptual basis

In the same way that nurses' values affect the nursing care received by patients, assessment instruments operationalize the author's perspective on nursing assessment. Therefore the conceptual basis specifies which theoretical approach is used to make the assessment and why, and also shows how the results obtained may be interpreted in light of that body of theory (McDowell and Newell 1987).

The conceptual basis of the assessment tools was addressed in only seven of the 22 studies reviewed. This is surprising, considering the prominence of nursing models in the literature and nurse education syllabi. There may be several possible reasons for this:

- a conceptual basis is not perceived as necessary for assessment guides for single constructs (interestingly all four of the studies involving multiple constructs within patient assessment describe the conceptual basis of the tool)
- many of the assessment tools are developed from practice experience and models are not well integrated into clinical practice settings
- purpose and conceptual basis of assessment tools are not differentiated so conceptual basis is assumed

- the intention of the assessment tool is to describe the patient's condition and therefore explaining the patient's condition in terms of the theory chosen is not considered necessary.

The conceptual basis in some of the studies reviewed was more developed than in others. Murphy and Moller (1993) based their tool to assess psychiatric symptoms on the Murphy Wellness Model, which describes the equilibrium between wellness and ill health and the factors that affect this. Similarly, Davis (1989) draws on themes of chronic pain, focusing specifically on the personal response to living with pain. In both these studies, results were explained in light of the conceptual basis and these were strengthened as a consequence. However, in some studies, the conceptual basis was not clearly explained, e.g. Chang et al. (1988) and Nokes et al. (1994), and its contribution to the explanation of the findings is unclear. Tettero et al. (1993) and Carboni (1992) both use Rogers (1970) Science of Unitary Beings as a conceptual framework. However, Rogers's theory is not well accepted in the UK and its contribution to patient assessment is poorly understood.

Method of assessment tool development

Although four of the studies reviewed did not specify how the tools were developed, great similarities were found in the studies that did discuss this. Common strategies used were:

- review of existing literature
- experience of authors
- and expert opinion.

Some of the studies used a combination of strategies. Frequently a literature search was conducted in the subject area to elicit the items for the tool, which was then scrutinized by a panel of experts who judged its comprehensiveness and the appropriateness of each item. Of the six studies that specified that items on the assessment tool were generated from the literature, none specified the parameters of the search in detail, e.g. types of texts, the source of the search, how literature was selected. Therefore the comprehensiveness of the literature found had to be assumed. Guidance on how items were generated from the literature would have been helpful.

In the nine studies that used expert opinion to develop the assessment tool, the number of experts used and the rationale for what constitutes an expert varied considerably. The number of experts used ranged from three (Blaylock and Cason 1992) to 45 (Hurley et al. 1992), with a few studies not specifying. Little guidance was found regarding what constitutes an appropriate number of experts. Waltz et al. (1991) suggested that it depended on the type of procedure, a point on which they did not elaborate. However, they did specify that an expert should be conversant with the domain treated in the assessment tool, and suggested that appropriate criteria to guide the selection of individuals with expertise should be identified. Again studies varied considerably in the way this was addressed. A few did not specify what they considered an expert to be, while other studies were detailed. Algase and Beel-Bates (1993) selected experts who were listed in the *Directory of Nurse Researchers* (Sigma Theta Tau 1987) under cognition, memory, mental status, confusion/disorientation and wandering, and who had a related article indexed in Cumulative Index of Nursing and Allied Health literature between 1983 and 1987.

Not all the studies reviewed generated tool items from the literature. Some sought information from the experience of clinical practice. In developing their tool to assess discomfort in patients with Alzheimers disease, Hurley et al. (1992) interviewed 45 nurses of all grades who worked in units specializing in the care of patients with Alzheimer's disease. In a similar way, Crandall and Getchell-Reiter (1993) developed a guide for sepsis in neonates using in-depth interviews with practising nurses to elicit assessment parameters and cognitive factors specific to clinical judgement. Interestingly, some discrepancy was found between expert opinion and published literature. Crandall and Getchell-Reiter (1993) found many differences between indicators of sepsis described in medical and nursing texts and indicators described by experienced nurses. Similarly WCCNR (1991) found that expert judgement differed from the literature. In this situation, does one form of judgement take precedence over the other? Although the discrepancy was acknowledged by both the studies above, they did not address whether there was a need to resolve it.

Psychometric characteristics of instruments

> An ideal measuring instrument is one that results in measures that are relevant, accurate, unbiased, sensitive, unidimensional and efficient.
>
> Polit and Hungler (1987)

These criteria are rather stringent and it is very unlikely that any assessment tools match this ideal. In classic measurement theory, an observed score in any measure is seen as a combination of a true score (what the subject would get if the instrument were perfect) and random and systematic error. Random error results from chance variations in the process of measurement. The amount of random error is inversely related to the degree of reliability of the measuring instrument (Carmines and Zeller 1979). Systematic or non-random error results from the presence of extraneous factors that affect all measurements made with the tool in the same way. Systematic bias compromises validity, the extent to which an instrument measures what it intends to measure.

Reliability and validity testing of a measuring instrument are crucial to indicate the degree of confidence that can be placed in any subsequent judgements or relationships using the tool.

Reliability

A vital characteristic that any instrument must possess is reliability (Jacobson 1992). Essentially the reliability of an instrument is the degree of consistency or repeatability with which it measures the attribute it is supposed to be measuring. The reliability of a measuring tool can be assessed in several different ways depending on the nature of the instrument and the aspect of the reliability concept that is of greatest interest. Polit and Hungler (1987) identify three aspects of reliability: stability, equivalence and internal consistency. It is often possible and desirable to use more than one approach.

Reliability as stability

The stability of a measure depends on the degree to which the same results are obtained when the instrument is administered repeatedly. Here, the focus of the reliability estimation is the instrument's susceptibility to the influence of extraneous factors from one administration to the next (Polit and Hungler 1987). Assessment of the stability of a measuring instrument is derived through test-retest reliability techniques. This involves administering the same test to the same sample of individuals on two separate occasions and correlating the scores obtained. While the test-retest method is relatively straightforward to use, it does have disadvantages. The first is that many attributes of interest do change over time, independently of the measure, due to intervening experiences between the two testings. Also the response on the second testing may be influenced by memory of response made on the first test and finally subjects may actually change in some way, e.g. attitudes or behaviours as a result of the first administration of the test. Therefore this method is best suited to more enduring characteristics that are thought to be unlikely to change easily. The time between administration of tests must be carefully considered.

Of the 22 studies reviewed, only four discussed test-retest reliability. Holmes and Mountain (1993) decided that test-retest reliability was not appropriate to test oral assessment tools, as oral status may change rapidly even within hours. The time interval between administration of tests in the other three studies (McMillan and Williams 1989, Nokes et al. 1994 and Davis 1989) varied, and the rationale for the interval used was rarely explained. McMillan and Williams (1989) used a time interval of one hour, Davis (1989) of two weeks and with Nokes et al. (1994) the time interval varied from 24 hours in hospitalized patients with AIDS to one week in healthy subjects. The time interval of one hour in the McMillan and Williams study seems too short to exclude the influence of memory. Nokes et al. (1994) explained that the relatively brief time interval in hospitalized patients was necessary because substantial changes in symptoms were possible in this group of individuals in brief periods of time. However, this does suggest that test-retest reliability may not be appropriate for testing this scale. While Davis (1989) selected a more suitable time interval, the scale was administered under different conditions, which would introduce various extraneous factors that may affect responses. Both McMillan and Williams (1989) and Nokes (1994) used apparently healthy adults, which would seem unsuitable since neither tool was designed to be used with healthy adults. Therefore the test-retest reliability assessments in the studies reviewed must be questioned for accuracy.

Reliability as equivalence

Reliability as equivalence has two forms. Both forms aim to determine the consistency or equivalence of the instrument in yielding measurements of the same characteristics in the same subjects. Parallel forms reliability requires the development of two different tests that measure the same trait or attribute in the same way. This procedure overcomes the problem of memory involvement associated with test-retest reliability. However, it is not commonly used in nursing research because of the difficulty in constructing parallel tests (Polit and Hungler 1987). The second form of reliability as equivalence is inter-rater reliability. This has been defined by Polit and Hungler (1987) as 'when different observers or researchers are using an instrument to measure the same phenomenon at the same time'. The potential weakness of inter-rater reliability is the fallibility of the researcher. Polit and Hungler (1987) suggest that careful training in how to use the measurement tool and the development of clearly defined, non-overlapping categories can increase the accuracy of later measurements and thus improve inter-rater reliability.

Of the studies reviewed, none used the parallel forms method to test reliability. Inter-rater reliability testing was the most frequently used form of reliability testing, with nine studies using this method. In some of the studies, the procedure used to collect data for inter-rater reliability was not described (WCCNR 1991, Mayer et al. 1989, Blaylock and Cason 1992, Fielding and Rowley 1990), which does not allow the method of testing to be examined. In the other studies, the raters tended to collect data simultaneously and score independently. Can two assessors truly assess a patient at the same time without influencing each other? The studies of Hurley et al. (1992), Miller (1990) and Holmes and Mountain (1993) all involve observation of patient condition where the independence of two assessors in their rating would seem to be more possible. However, the raters in McMillan et al. (1988) used a pain assessment tool simultaneously, which involved questioning the patient in areas such as 'Describe in your own words what your pain feels like'. In this situation, independent assessment seems unlikely. Chang et al.'s (1988) assessment tool also involved patient interview, and to provide for independent assessment while minimizing the period during which clinical conditions may have changed, patients were assessed by different raters within two to four hours of each other.

Four of the studies used percentage agreement between raters to estimate reliability (McMillan et al. 1988, Mayer et al. 1989, Miller 1990 and Chang et al. 1988), even though this method tends to overestimate observer agreements because it does not take occurrence of agreement by chance into account (Polit and Hungler 1987). The other studies used correlation coefficients. However, Holmes and Mountain (1993) perceived a discrepancy between the high correlation between the total scores of raters and marked differences in scoring of categories within the scales. Chang et al. (1988) questioned whether low inter-rater reliability for some items was due to the instrument itself, changes in the patient in the two to four hours between assessments or lack of explicit definitions regarding some of the observations and judgements required by the nurse. Miller (1990) found inter-rater reliability of incontinence assessments to be high and this she attributed to intensive training. To conclude, the estimates of inter-rater reliability were not well reported and those reported showed inconsistencies.

Reliability as internal consistency

Internal consistency is the extent to which subparts or items of an instrument are all measuring the same attribute or dimension and nothing else. The internal consistency approach to estimating an instrument's reliability is thought by Polit and Hungler (1987) to be the most widely used method.

One method of assessing internal consistency is the split-half technique, where the items of a single test are divided into halves, usually odd- and even-numbered items, scored separately and a correlation coefficient of the two halves calculated. However, the correlation coefficient computed on split halves of a measure tends to underestimate the reliability of the entire scale. Although the split-half technique is easy to use, its chief disadvantage is that different reliability estimates can be obtained by using different 'splits'. To compensate for this deficiency, internal consistency is increasingly being estimated by use of statistical formulae. The preferred method being the Chronbach coefficient alpha (Jacobson 1992), which gives an estimate of the split-half correlation for all possible ways of dividing the individual item scores of the measure into two halves.

Five of the studies reviewed examined internal consistency as an estimate of reliability. None of these studies used the split-half technique, all used the Chronbach coefficient alpha (Crosby and Parsons 1989, McMillan and Williams 1989, Nokes et al. 1994, Davis 1989 and Algase and Beel-Bates 1993). Interestingly, Davis used alpha coefficient to refine the items of an instrument to measure chronic pain and discard items that were not contributing to the internal consistency. However, details of the procedures used to do this were not reported.

Validity

The second vital characteristic of the quality of a measuring instrument is validity. Polit and Hungler (1987) define validity as 'the degree to which an instrument measures what it is supposed to be measuring'. In a similar way to reliability, there are several different aspects of validity and approaches of assessment. However, unlike reliability, validity is very difficult to establish. Reliability of an instrument is a prerequisite of validity (Polit and Hungler 1987). This is because an unreliable or inconsistent tool is likely to be measuring too many other factors associated with random error to be measuring the attribute of interest accurately. While the literature identifies many types of validity, Polit and Hungler (1987) classify three: content, criterion-related and construct validity. Jacobson (1992) adds a fourth, face validity, and therefore these four will be discussed here.

Face validity

Face validity is the weakest form of validity (Fox 1982), involving a judgement of what the tool appears to measure based on lay opinion (Jacobson 1992). It provides no evidence of what the tool is really measuring. Of the studies reviewed, only one addressed face validity (Nokes et al. 1994). Since this tool aimed to assess HIV-related symptom severity and general wellbeing, checking relevance of the items in the tool with potential respondents may increase its acceptability.

Content validity

Content validity refers to whether or not the test items comprehensively represent the content area being measured. There are no objective methods of assuring adequate content coverage of an instrument and therefore content validity is based on judgement. This judgement is commonly based on the consensus of experts in the content area (Polit and Hungler 1987). An index of content validity (CVI) showing the proportion of agreement between judges can be computed (Waltz et al. 1991). Consensus of opinion in existing literature is also useful way of establishing content validity (Jacobson 1992). Polit and Hungler (1987) consider that the careful consideration and specification of the attribute and how it can be measured is important in demonstrating content validity. Of the studies reviewed, ten discussed content validity. The most common method used was that of expert judgement (eight studies), with three of these computing a content validity index as described by Waltz et al. (1991). As previously discussed, few of the studies identified how experts were selected and on what criteria they were asked to judge the tools which would justify their claim for content validity. Three studies claimed satisfactory content validity on the basis of congruence with the literature reviewed, the comprehensiveness of which was not demonstrated.

Criterion-related validity

Criterion-related validity of an instrument is demonstrated if scores correlate highly with an appropriate external criterion. The availability of a reasonably reliable and valid criterion with which to compare the measures on the target instrument is crucial, but unfortunately is difficult to attain. Two types of criterion-related validity are commonly distinguished. Concurrent validity is concerned with the instrument's ability to discriminate between individuals who differ in their present status on some criterion. Predictive validity, on the other hand, refers to the extent an instrument can predict the respondent's behaviour or performance on some criterion observed at a future time. Fox (1982) suggested that tool users should demand evidence of predictive validity in clinical tools, although this was not addressed in any of the studies reviewed.

Waltz et al. (1991) considered criterion-related validity to be the most pertinent when a tool will be used for decision making. It is therefore surprising that only four of the studies reviewed addressed the issue of criterion-related validity, since a majority purport to aid assessment on which care decisions are made. Although Chang et al. (1988) acknowledged the desirability of obtaining a measure of criterion validity, known and valid external criteria were not available. This is possibly the reason why other studies do not report criterion-related validity even though it would seem to be appropriate.

Explanation of why a criterion is appropriate is important and should be made explicit (Knapp 1985). Blaylock and Cason (1992) did not explain why they used patient age and length of stay as criteria to estimate validity of a discharge planning risk tool even though they may also be aspects of other constructs, for example multiple pathology, type and severity of disease, duration of treatment used. Similarly Nokes et al. (1994) did not specify why a modified Karnofsky scale was selected as an objective measure of quality of life as a criterion to estimate the validity of their HIV-related symptom severity and general wellbeing scale.

Waltz et al. (1991) insisted that prior to using predictor and criterion measures in criterion-related validity studies, each should have demonstrated sufficient evidence for reliability and validity, a requirement neglected in all three studies addressing criterion-related validity. Nokes et al. did not report reliability or validity evidence for the Karnofsky scale; Crosby and Parsons (1989) relied on published evidence of reliability and validity of the Glasgow coma scale, which may not be appropriate to their sample or assessors; and Brians et al. (1991) failed to test their falls risk assessment tool prior to correlating the scores with incidence of subsequent falls.

Construct validity

Construct validity is concerned with the question of what the tool is actually measuring, and is very difficult to substantiate. The importance of construct validity lies in its link with theory and theoretical conceptualization, and therefore there is always an emphasis on logical analysis and the testing of relationships predicted on the basis of theoretical propositions. The concept being measured is seen as part of a network of associated concepts and meanings (a construct), which enables the researcher to predict how one construct will function in relation to other constructs.

Construct validity can be approached in several ways. In known-groups technique, the instrument is administered to two groups expected to differ on the key attribute because of some other known characteristic. If the groups' scores differ significantly, construct validity is supported. Another method to examine construct validity is the multitrait-multimethod matrix method. This procedure is based on the concepts of convergence and discriminality. Convergence is demonstrated by evidence that different methods of measuring a construct give similar results. Discriminality refers to the ability of an instrument to differentiate the construct being measured from other similar constructs. Scores from at least two constructs, each measured in at least two different ways, are entered into a correlation matrix from which separate correlations indicating discriminant and convergent validity can be obtained. The third method commonly used is factor analysis. This is a complex mathematical method that identifies clusters of related variables. Each cluster or factor represents one attribute. Factor analysis can be used to identify whether a concept is unidimensional or multidimensional, depending on whether one or several factors are needed to describe it. Essentially factor analysis is another means of examining convergent and discriminant validity.

Seven of the studies reviewed addressed construct validity. Three of these used known-groups technique. McMillan and Williams (1989) claimed that the significantly different results between patients with cancer being treated with neurotoxic chemotherapeutic agents or regular morphine and normal healthy adults supported the construct validity of the constipation assessment scale. However, Waltz et al. (1991) warned that the difference in scores on an instrument may be due to non-comparability in another variable that was not measured, and that a claim of validity must be offered in light of this possibility. While it may seem unlikely that the constipation assessment scale is measuring anything else, there may be differences other than constipation between a group of patients being treated for cancer and a group of normal healthy adults. A better group comparison was used to examine the scale's ability to differentiate constipation intensity. For this, patients who had not received a dose of neurotoxic chemotherapy for three weeks and were expected to have milder symptoms were compared with patients currently receiving substantial doses of morphine.

To examine the construct validity of their Pain Flow Sheet (PFS), McMillan et al. (1988) looked at whether it fulfilled its purpose as a tool to aid pain management by documenting nursing plans, actions and patient outcomes. They claimed that the significantly lower pain intensity experienced when the PFS was used supported its construct validity. However, reliability testing had not been done and without this these results were unsubstantiated. Hurley et al. (1992) compared the discomfort scores of patients during the peak of a fever episode, which is presumed to cause discomfort, with the patients' baseline score as a sign of construct validity.

Although none of the studies reviewed claimed to use multitrait-multimethod procedures, three discussed convergent and discriminant validity. Nokes et al. (1994) tested the discriminant validity of their HIV assessment tool by comparing the scores of HIV-positive groups with the healthy groups and people with AIDS. WCCNR (1991) correlated the scores of their stomatitis staging system with the Oral Assessment Guide (OAG) and the World Health Organisation (WHO) Mucositis Grading Scale to test for convergent validity. However, the researchers relied on former reliability testing of these instruments, which is not ideal. Algase and Beel-Bates (1993) found that their Everyday Indication of Impaired Cognition (EIIC) scale correlated to the Memory-Orientation-Concentration (MOC) test and the Mini Mental Status Examination (MMSE) at values to support convergent validity. Divergent validity was supported by the small, non-significant correlations of the EIIC with the Bradburn Affect Balance Scale (ABS). Again evidence of reliability of the MOC, MMSE and ABS was taken from former studies.

Only two studies used a factor analysis procedure. Algase and Beel-Bates (1993) used it to develop and refine their assessment tool, although they did not overtly use the data to support construct validity. Davis (1989) used factor analysis and predictive modeling, a procedure that is beyond the scope of this review, to test construct validity. It was the only study reviewed that actually linked the findings of the study to existing theory and discussed the implications, which was disappointing since this is a specific consideration of construct validity. The other studies focused on the assessment tool development per se.

Conclusion

It can be seen from this review that the construction and evaluation of assessment tools is a complex issue. Although the studies reviewed did not have contents similar to that of the NLIU physical assessment framework, the exploration of methods of developing assessment tools has highlighted many areas of difficulty that will be taken into account when the NLIU framework is examined and tested. Unfortunately the studies generally did not give reasons for the decisions made in the methodology, and while this may have been due to the length of the general reports, it does limit conclusions that can be drawn from them.

From the review of literature concerning nurses' assessment, it is suggested that the use of assessment tools designed for specific use in practice settings would considerably improve nurses' assessment of patients. As an assessment tool developed in a clinical practice area, the NLIU physical assessment framework has the potential to be a useful tool to improve nursing practice. In Chapter 2, it will be critically explored in terms of its purpose, conceptual basis and development.

Chapter 2
Development and refinement of the Byron Physical Assessment Framework

This chapter critically explores the Byron Physical Assessment Framework (BPAF), starting with the history of the tool and the circumstances of its development. The remainder of the chapter discusses the BPAF under the headings 'Description', 'Purpose', 'Conceptual basis' and 'How developed', which were used to structure the review of existing assessment tools in the previous chapter (McDowell and Newell 1987). Reliability and validity are dealt with in separate chapters.

Aims and objectives

This initial phase was intended to fulfil the first aim of the study: 'To examine the content and conceptual basis for the assessment framework and make any necessary changes to refine it'. To do this, the following objectives were set:

- To review and describe the initial development, conceptual basis and purpose of the BPAF
- To examine the content of the BPAF and revise as necessary to improve its comprehensiveness and clarity for its intended purpose.

Description of the nursing-led inpatient unit

In February 1993, the Nursing Development Unit (NDU) established a nursing-led inpatient unit (NLIU) for medical inpatients, whereby medically stable patients with significant nursing needs are transferred to the care of a primary nurse who takes full responsibility for co-ordinating the remainder of the patients hospital stay. (The NLIU was established and developed as part of the NDU. From this point the unit will be referred to as the NLIU for simplicity, although it was always part of the NDU.) As their hospital stay progresses, the focus of many patients' needs changes from technical medical intervention involving diagnosis and treatment of an acute crisis, to care related to rehabilitation and education. The Audit Commission 1992 report *Lying in Wait* considered that 48% of patients in acute medical beds did not require acute medical services although still requiring inpatient care. Generally these patients remain in acute wards, where the priority for nursing must be the management of acute crisis. Therefore by transferring these patients to the NLIU the acute wards can concentrate on the needs of the acutely ill and the NLIU can focus on the changed needs of the patient.

Medical cover is still required for these patients even though their care is led by the primary nurse. Non-urgent, day-to-day medical intervention is provided by a rheumatology registrar employed on a sessional basis. Cover for a medical emergency is provided by the on-call acute medical team. Specialist medical consultation is requested by the nurses within the normal referral mechanisms. Should a patient become medically unstable, the patient is referred back to the original consultant physician who will decide whether or not to move the patient to an acute bed. A more detailed description of this service can be found in Evans and Griffiths (1994).

History of the BPAF

While the establishment of the nursing-led service provided the final impetus to develop the BPAF, the NDU had already recognized the need for a more systematized assessment process. During a documentation audit in 1992, several problems with assessment were identified (Batehup and Evans 1992). These included:

- absence of evidence of continued patient assessment
- absence of evidence of continued assessment of identified problems, with the exception of where a structured assessment format was used, for example in pain and wound management
- difficulty in gaining an overall picture of a patient's condition and identifying trends over time.

The establishment of the NLIU introduced new responsibilities for nursing. While medical stability is one of the criteria for patient suitability for the nursing-led service, it was recognized to be a transient phenomenon. Therefore it was deemed essential for nursing staff to systematically review their patients each day to detect any changes in their physical condition and arrange timely medical input during one of the Unit doctor's four two-hour sessions each week. To facilitate this, remedy problems identified by Batehup and Evans, and fulfil the statutory requirement to document nursing assessment, the BPAF was developed by the nursing staff.

Purpose of the BPAF

The BPAF gives structure to assessment to enable nurses to make a comprehensive assessment of the patient's physical condition, focusing on a wide range of physiological abnormalities. It was designed to be used with patients suitable for the NLIU, i.e. adults whose acute medical crisis has resolved but who still have health needs which are best met with intensive nursing therapy. However, its content is very general and therefore it is likely to be applicable to other patient groups as well.

On the NLIU it is used in two circumstances:

- As a daily assessment to monitor the patient's physical condition. Each day a member of qualified staff is required to assess the patient using the BPAF. Any new abnormal findings should be assessed further and documented in the medical notes, with details of action taken and referrals made to other health professionals. Using the BPAF in this way is believed to detect deterioration in a patient's condition at the earliest possible stage to enable timely intervention by the unit doctor to prevent the occurrence of an acute medical crisis.
- As part of the procedure to screen suitable patients referred to the NLIU according to the Unit's criteria (Evans and Griffiths 1994). The use of the BPAF is intended to provide a detailed baseline of the patient's physical condition and to identify any physical problems that may have appeared since the last detailed medical assessment and which may need medical attention prior to transfer, should the patient be considered suitable to be cared for in the NLIU.

The BPAF is not designed to guide nurses to diagnose medical problems, as this was considered to be inappropriate and beyond the scope of their role. However, it is designed to enable nurses to identify and articulate deviations from the patient's norm in a more specific and systematic way. This is particularly important in a NLIU where, unlike on the acute wards, gaining medical attention for a patient is formally dependent on nursing initiation and requires a far more structured assessment of the patient in order to make informed and coherent referrals. Thus the BPAF was one of the important 'safety nets' initiated by the unit to ensure that all patient needs were met and that adjustment of the NDU's 'scope of professional practice' was not 'detrimental to the interests, condition or safety of patients' (UKCC 1992).

This structured daily documentation of the assessment of a patient's physical condition also begins to address some of the problems in assessment documentation identified by Batehup and Evans (1992) by enabling trends in patient condition to emerge and providing information about a patient that does not necessarily constitute a problem requiring a nursing care plan.

Conceptual basis of the BPAF

The BPAF is based on physiological body systems and involves the collection of data concerning patients' physical signs and symptoms to enable the detection of abnormalities and initiation of appropriate treatment and referral to resolve and stabilize those abnormal findings. Therefore the BPAF fits most neatly into the so-called 'medical model', whereby abnormal body function is investigated to discover a diagnosis which indicates the most appropriate treatment to cure the underlying disease causing the abnormal symptoms. However, while the medical model has been very successful in treating pathological disease, its focus is often criticized as being narrow and reductionist leading to fragmentation of care and the exclusion of consideration of psychological and sociological factors that influence health (Holden 1990). Possibly in response to this, many nursing models concentrate on psychological and sociological factors. Reed and Watson (1994) argue that nurses may be replacing physiological reductionism with psychological reductionism in an attempt to distance themselves from the medical profession and establish nursing as an independent profession.

Although the conceptual basis of the BPAF is primarily derived from the medical model and the need to be proactive in meeting patient needs rather than reactive once an acute crisis has occurred, it must be emphasized that the BPAF is only part of the nursing assessment. Assessment of nursing needs and care planning is conducted according to a format loosely based on the work of Roper et al. (1980), whereby the goal of nursing care is to restore the patient to his or her previous level of independence or, where this is not possible, to help the patient cope with a reduced level of independence. In line with the critique described by Walsh (1991), the ward team had previously added categories of emotional wellbeing, pain, educational needs and social situation to the lifestyle assessment documentation incorporating Roper et al.'s 12 activities of living.

Description of the BPAF

The BPAF in use at the beginning of this study was a 50-item checklist comprised of five body systems:

- oxygenation
- food and fluid
- elimination
- skin
- neurological (see Appendix 2 for complete version).

Each of these sections is compiled of signs and symptoms of abnormal physiology appropriate to each system. Some of the signs are starred, e.g. respiratory rate, pulse rate and special diet/feeding requiring the nurse to document values. A majority of items require the nurse to sign against any abnormal signs or symptoms assessed. These items are judged to be either absent or present. The BPAF does not differentiate between degree or severity of abnormal signs or symptoms. In the presence of new abnormal findings, the nursing staff are required to assess the abnormality further and document their assessment in the medical notes together with subsequent action taken (see Figure 2.1).

		M	T	W	T	F	S	S
O **X** **Y**	Respiration: rate (normal 12-18)* laboured other abnormality	15	1 6	20 AE				
G **E** **N** **A**	Cough Sputum Moist Wheeze			AE AE AE				

T **I** **O** **N**	Pulse: rate*
	    irregular
	    weak
	 Chest pain
	 Pitting oedema
	 Calf pain
	 Dizziness on standing							

Medical notes entry: *Chest sounding moist, patient complains of productive cough - yellow sputum. Respiratory rate 20 breaths/min and is laboured. Apyrexial. Sputum specimen sent for microscopy, culture and sensitivity. Medical review requested.*

(Evans and Griffiths 1994)

Figure 2.1. The use of the oxygenation section of the BPAF.

Development of the BPAF

The initial development of the BPAF was conducted by a small group of ward staff as part of the preparation work for establishing nursing-led beds. Ideas for an alternative documentation format had already been considered (Batehup and Evans 1992). A structured flow sheet format was chosen as it was considered to be easy to complete and time saving, and it enables trends in patient condition to be easily identified (Iyer and Camp 1995). Ideas for how to format the flow sheet were taken from the PIE system designed by Siegrist et al. (1985), although the content was determined by the nurses' experience. The resultant flow sheet (see Appendix 3) was in use from February 1993 to June 1994, when it was updated to the version previously described. The main reason for revision was to include physiological indicators of nursing care, data that were needed in the preliminary evaluation of the NLIU. These physiological indicators of nursing care were taken from Majesky et al. (1978), whose work to devise a tool to measure quality of nursing care resulted in the identification of observable physiological indicators of negative patient outcomes which represent nursing accountable complications. These indicators are signs of infection, immobility and fluid imbalance. Some of the indicators were already present in the original BPAF, i.e. altered chest sounds, respiratory rate, hard stool and loose stool. Indicators that were added are:

- sputum
- calf pain
- dizziness on standing
- reduced tissue turgor
- dry mouth
- coated mouth
- weekly weight
- concentrated urine
- body temperature
- reddening of pressure areas
- ulceration/damage
- purulent wound
- contracture/spasticity.

Other items not cited by Majesky et al. were also added to increase the comprehensiveness of the BPAF in assessing physical condition. These are:

- pulse rate
- nausea
- poor appetite
- dysphagia
- special diet feeding
- presence of a urinary catheter
- having separate items for central and peripheral cyanosis.

A major difference between the two versions was that the original version had normal physiological states included in the item list and abnormal symptoms were in bold boxes indicating a requirement for action (see Figure 2.2 and compare with Figure 2.1).

After revision the BPAF was more comprehensive and addressed aspects of physical condition not previously included. The BPAF now assessed acute deterioration of patient condition treated by nursing intervention in addition to deterioration treated by medical intervention.

Both versions of the BPAF have been well accepted by the ward staff, who report that they felt their assessment of patients had become more systematic and comprehensive through its use. In a series of interviews conducted by a project development nurse during 1993, medical staff were appreciative of the assessment skills of the NLIU nurses when asking for medical assistance. As one doctor commented:

R E S P	Unlaboured								
	Laboured								
	Other abnormality								
	Rate: normal (12-18)								
	rapid								
	Sounds: clear								
	moist								
	cough								
	stridor								
	wheeze								
C I R C	Pulse: regular								
	irregular								
	strong								
	weak								
	Chest pain								
	Pitting oedema								

Figure 2.2. The respiration and circulation sections of the original version of the BPAF.

> they will usually have done a brief assessment ... might have thought about sending some initial bloods tests off, sometimes these will have been done ... they're more confident. They'll look at the patient as a whole and see whether they're symptomatic, whether they've got headaches or whatever in the case of high blood pressure so they'll be less alarmist.
>
> Cited in Griffiths and Evans (1995)

To evaluate the effectiveness of the NLIU, a randomized controlled study has been conducted comparing clinical outcomes of patients cared for on the NLIU with patients cared for on the acute medical wards. An interim report (Griffiths and Evans 1995) shows that patients cared for on the NLIU were:

- more likely to be discharged to their own homes
- less physically dependent at discharge
- less likely to develop a pressure sore
- less likely to be diagnosed as having a chest infection or urinary tract infection.

While these results have been reported with caution until the replication study is completed, they still ask the crucial question of what happens on the unit that influences clinical outcomes. Griffiths and Evans did not offer any possible explanations. However, anecdotal suggestions from the nursing staff on the unit include the regular, comprehensive assessment facilitated by the BPAF.

The development of the BPAF has been haphazard. Its initial conception was based on the experience of ward nurses and its revision was largely based on Majesky et al.'s work, and it had not been tested in any way. Therefore to see whether the tool did affect the nurses' actions and thus was worth examining and developing further, a small preliminary investigation of the medical notes of past patients was conducted.

Preliminary investigation of the utilization of the BPAF

The aim of the preliminary investigation was to examine completed physical assessments using the BPAF and determine the action taken by the nursing staff as a result of a new abnormality being detected.

Method

A sample of 100 new abnormalities assessed by a nurse using the BPAF were sought from the medical notes of former NLIU patients selected using tables of random numbers generated by a computer. All patients had consented to be part of the research evaluating the NLIU, which involved giving permission for access to medical notes by a member of the NDU research team. During this study, the author had an honorary contract with the NDU as part of the research team.

For each set of notes scrutinized, the BPAFs were retrieved and inspected for the occurrence of new abnormalities assessed. Five consecutive abnormalities were selected and the action taken as a result of each assessment was found by examining the medical notes, the nursing notes and the unit doctor's communication book, where requests for medical review or other queries are recorded. To select the five consecutive newly identified abnormalities within each set of notes, the total number of new abnormalities that were assessed during the patient's stay on the NLIU were counted. To ensure that sampling extended over the whole length of stay and to remove the possibility of bias selection, a systematic approach was taken. The first five consecutive new abnormalities were selected from the first set of notes examined, then the second five new abnormalities were selected from the second set of notes examined, and so on.

The action taken in response to assessment of a new abnormal sign or symptom was assigned to one of three categories:

- no documentation/no action taken
- findings documented/action taken
- referral made to unit doctor, referring medical team or other member of the multidisciplinary team.

For some actions more than one category was used.

Results

Of the 100 new abnormalities assessed, 37% were referred for medical input. Thirty one percent were referred to the unit doctor, 7% were referred back to the referring medical team and 4% were seen by an on-call senior house officer (SHO) for urgent medical input. Some patients were referred for more than one type of medical input at the same time (e.g. unit doctor and referring medical team). Of the 31 referrals to the unit doctor, 18 required medical investigation and/or treatment. All the referrals back to the referring medical team resulted in the team taking some action, whether transferring the patient back to an acute ward or changing the medical treatment. Twenty nine percent of all new abnormalities assessed were documented by nursing staff either in the medical or nursing notes, and in some cases action was taken to investigate, e.g. take urine sample or electrocardiogram (ECG).

Overall, 59% of new abnormalities assessed via the BPAF were acted on in some way by the nursing staff, which would indicate that the BPAF does have some influence on the actions of the nursing staff and is thus worthy of further scrutiny and evaluation.

Refinement of the BPAF

Two methodologies were used to refine the BPAF, extensive literature review and expert opinion, as this appeared to be the most successful strategy used to develop assessment tools in the studies reviewed in Chapter 1. The aim was to examine the content, comprehensiveness, clarity, relevance, format and ease of use.

Literature review

To review the content of the BPAF, an extensive review of medical texts on physical examination was carried out (see Table 2.1). These texts were thought to be the most appropriate because the tool is based on physiological systems and they were selected on the advice of a lecturer responsible for a post-registration physical assessment module.

Table 2.1. Physical assessment texts selected for review

Author	Title
Munro and Edwards (1990)	Macleod's Clinical Examination
Bates (1995)	A Pocket Guide to Physical Examination and History Taking
Toghill (ed) (1995)	Examining Patients: an introduction to clinical medicine
Hayes and MacWalter (1992)	Aids to Clinical Examination
Turner and Blackwood (1991)	Lecture Notes on History Taking and Examination

To make examination easier, a table was compiled for each physiological system containing all the abnormal signs and symptoms described by each of the medical texts. The signs and symptoms already contained in the BPAF appear in bold type. Table 2.2 shows the respiratory system table. The other tables addressing the cardiovascular system, neurological system, gastrointestinal system and genitourinary system can be found in Appendices 4 to 7 respectively. The medical texts were also used to compile detailed definitions of each of the items on the BPAF and guidelines on how to conduct the assessment of each item (see Table 2.3; a full copy can be found in Appendix 8).

Table 2.2. Abnormal signs and symptoms of the respiratory system

	Munro and Edwards (1990)	Toghill (1995)	Bates (1995)	Turner and Blackwood (1991)	Hayes and MacWalter (1992)
Principal symptoms	6 specified (first 6 items)	3 specified (first 3 items)	none specified	none specified	none specified
Symptoms and signs of abnormal function (those in bold are items on the BPAF before this study. Those in italics are those added during the study)	- **dyspnoea** - **cough** - **chest pain** - **sputum** - *haemoptysis* - **wheeze** - *stridor* - **cyanosis central peripheral** - *abnormal chest wall movement* - abnormal appearance of chest wall - abnormal breath sounds on auscultation, e.g. diminished vesicular, bronchial, intermediate - *added breath sounds, e.g.* **rhonchi (wheezes), crepitations (crackles),** *pleural rub*	- **breathlessness** - **cough** - **chest pain** - **sputum** - *haemoptysis* - **wheeze** - *stridor* - **cyanosis central peripheral** - abnormal chest wall appearance - *abnormal chest wall movement* - abnormal breath sounds on auscultation, e.g. reduced, normal, bronchial - *added breath sounds* e.g **wheeze, crackles** *pleural rub* - *abnormal shape of chest wall* - abnormal percussion of chest	- **tachypnoea (rate)** - *hyperpnoea (effort)* - *irregular breathing pattern* - **abnormal depth of breathing** - shape of chest, e.g. barrel - *abnormal chest wall movement* - abnormal percussion of chest, e.g. hyper-resonance, dull - abnormal breath sounds, e.g. decreased breath sounds, bronchial, bronchovesicular - *added breath sounds, e.g.* **crackles (fine or course), wheezes or rhonchi** - abnormal transmitted breath sounds	- **abnormal respiratory rate** - **hypoxia** - hypercapnia - *irregular respiratory pattern* - **effort of breathing** - **wheeze** - abnormal shape of chest - *unequal movement of chest* - abnormal percussion of chest, eg. increased or decreased resonance - abnormal breath sounds on auscultation, e.g. bronchial, reduced breath sounds - *added breath sounds, e.g. pleural*	- **cyanosis, central and peripheral** - **breathlessness** - **use of accessory muscles of respiration** - abnormal shape of chest - *abnormal chest wall movement* - **abnormal respiratory rate** - *abnormal respiratory pattern* - **sputum** - abnormal percussion of chest, e.g. increased or decreased resonance - abnormal breath sounds on auscultation, e.g. bronchial, diminished

(contd)

Table 2.2. (contd)

	Munro and Edwards (1990)	Toghill (1995)	Bates (1995)	Turner and Blackwood (1991)	Hayes and MacWalter (1992)
		e.g hyper-resonance dull, stony dull - abnormal transmission of voice sounds - peak expiratory flow rate (PEFR)	NB Particularly concerned with the process of examination rather than the comprehensive findings	*rub*, **wheeze, crackles (fine - heart failure, medium - infection or coarse - bronchiectasis)** - abnormal voice resonance **- sputum** - abnormal PEFR	- *added breath sounds*, e.g. **crepitations, rhonchi,** *pleural rub* - abnormal voice resonance
Normal values **Respiratory rate**	14/min in healthy adult at rest	10-15/min >20 (very abnormal)	14-20/min in adults	no normal values given	no normal values given

Table 2.3. Extract from item definition table

Item on the BPAF	Definition
Pulse: rate	Generally the radial pulse is taken as a measurement of heart rate, although in some situations they may not be the same. Pulse rate value is generally assumed to denote number of heartbeats per minute. Pulse should be assessed over a minute to ensure that any irregularities and abnormalities have been assessed
irregular	Can be regularly or irregularly irregular. The normal pulse should be of regular, even rhythm and volume. Should the pulse be irregular in any way the apex beat should also be assessed for rate and rhythm and any deficit between the apex and radial beats determined
weak	Generally the pulse is said to be weak when it is difficult to palpate, i.e. the rise and fall of the blood vessel feels faint under the finger. Systolic BP of 50 mmHg is required to palpate a femoral or brachial pulse and needs to be higher to palpate a radial pulse

Expert group

A group of eight experts was used to examine the second version of the BPAF. They were selected on the basis that they had extensive knowledge on physical assessment or assessment tool development, or extensive experience using the BPAF. This was in line with Waltz et al.'s (1991) specification that an expert should be conversant with the domain treated in the assessment tool and that the criteria on which they were selected be identified (see Table 2.4).

Each of the experts was sent a copy of the BPAF, the tables of abnormal physiological signs and symptoms, and the item definitions and guidelines for assessment. An explanation of the purpose of the BPAF, its use on the NLIU and its conceptual basis was included with the request that they examine the tool's content in terms of comprehensiveness, clarity and relevance to intended purpose. They then met to discuss their thoughts. Each item and its definition were reviewed in turn and suggestions for improvement were discussed and agreed on. Signs and symptoms that were considered important to add to the BPAF were also discussed and a decision made as to whether to include them. The experts also looked at the format and the organization of items within the BPAF.

Table 2.4. Areas of applicable experience and expertise of experts used in the study

Job title	Area of applicable expertise/experience
Assessment nurse, NLIU	Assesses suitability of patients for NLIU. Has completed degree module in physical assessment. Experience of using BPAF
Assessment nurse, NLIU	Assesses suitability of patients for NLIU. Has completed degree module in physical assessment. Experience of using BPAF
Primary nurse, NLIU	Responsible for a caseload of 'nurse-led' patients. Experience of using BPAF
Clinical researcher, NLIU	Development of documentation audit tools. Has completed degree module in physical assessment. Experience of using BPAF
Unit doctor, NLIU	Clinical training focused on physical assessment
Lecturer	Responsible for post-registration degree module in physical assessment. MSc thesis on nurses' assessment of patients
Lecturer/ practitioner, acute medicine	Extensive experience in audit and development of audit tools
Researcher of this study	Formerly senior primary nurse/ward manager on the NDU with experience of using the BPAF

Changes made to the BPAF

A number of changes were made to the BPAF as a result of the review of medical texts and expert opinion. These are discussed under three headings: structure, content and changes in item definition. (See Figure 2.3 for the revised BPAF.)

Structure

The flow sheet format was considered appropriate and there were no suggestions to change this. Changes were made to the titles of systems to increase cohesion with the physiological systems represented. Oxygenation system was replaced with respiratory system and cardio-vascular system, similarly the food and fluid section was replaced with gastrointestinal system. Elimination system was replaced with urinary system, with bowel assessment being incorporated into gastrointestinal system. A section representing temperature was added. Some of the skin section items were considered better placed in other systems.

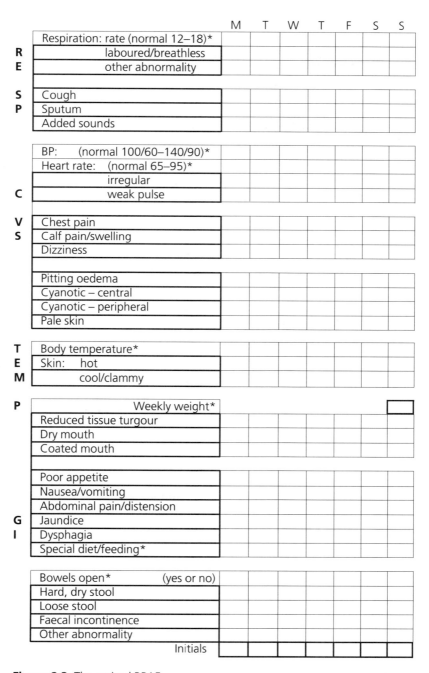

		M	T	W	T	F	S	S
R	Respiration: rate (normal 12–18)*							
E	laboured/breathless							
	other abnormality							
S	Cough							
P	Sputum							
	Added sounds							
	BP: (normal 100/60–140/90)*							
	Heart rate: (normal 65–95)*							
	irregular							
C	weak pulse							
V	Chest pain							
S	Calf pain/swelling							
	Dizziness							
	Pitting oedema							
	Cyanotic – central							
	Cyanotic – peripheral							
	Pale skin							
T	Body temperature*							
E	Skin: hot							
M	cool/clammy							
P	Weekly weight*							
	Reduced tissue turgour							
	Dry mouth							
	Coated mouth							
	Poor appetite							
	Nausea/vomiting							
	Abdominal pain/distension							
G	Jaundice							
I	Dysphagia							
	Special diet/feeding*							
	Bowels open* (yes or no)							
	Hard, dry stool							
	Loose stool							
	Faecal incontinence							
	Other abnormality							
	Initials							

Figure 2.3. The revised BPAF.

(contd)

Figure 2.3. (contd)

		M	T	W	T	F	S	S
U	Dysuria							
R	Frequency/urgency							
I	Concentrated urine							
N	Odour							
E	Incontinent							
	Catheterized							
N	Headache							
E	Visual disturbance							
U	Paraesthesiae							
R	Lethargic/mood change							
O	Disorientated/confused							
M	Slurred speech/dysarthric							
U	Dysphasic							
S	Limb: weakness/flaccid							
C	contracture/stiffness							
U	Joint/muscular pain							
L	Joint/tissue swelling							
A	Rash							
R	Reddening of pressure areas							
	Skin ulceration/damage							
	Purulent wound							
	Initials							

Figure 2.3. The revised BPAF.

Cyanosis was moved to the cardiovascular system, jaundice was moved to the gastrointestinal system and although pale fits into both cardiovascular and gastrointestinal systems, it was moved to the cardiovascular system. The remainder of the skin section, i.e. reddening of pressure areas, ulceration/damage and purulent wound was moved to the neuromuscular section, thus removing the skin section completely. It was suggested that for consistency, items that were symptoms should come before signs, in the same way that medical staff assess symptoms first. This was done as far as possible, although at times this principle was compromised to preserve cohesiveness within systems. An example of this can be seen in the cardiovascular system (see Figure 2.3). The vital signs in the system are listed first to give them prominence, and while 'irregular' and 'weak pulse' are signs, they were put next because they would have been assessed at the same time as heart rate.

Symptoms of 'chest pain', 'calf pain and swelling' and 'dizziness' come next, followed by the signs 'pitting oedema', 'cyanotic - central', 'cyanotic - peripheral' and 'pale skin'.

Content

There were some changes to the content of the BPAF. Generally these changes involved adding items or changing the wording of items to add clarity or extend scope. In the respiratory section, little was changed. The item 'laboured' was expanded to 'laboured/breathless', to include the patient's subjective feeling of difficulty breathing. 'Wheeze' and 'moist' were deleted and incorporated into 'added sounds'. There were more changes in the cardiovascular section. 'Blood pressure' was added because it was the only vital sign not included and is an important part of cardiovascular assessment. The normal ranges of values given for all vital signs are intentionally narrow, as many patients on the unit are elderly and their physical tolerance for abnormal vital signs is lower than that of younger people. 'Pulse' was substituted by 'heart rate' as a more accurate term. 'Dizziness on standing' was changed to 'dizziness', to include any occurrence of dizziness. Some changes were made to the gastrointestinal system. 'Nausea' was expanded to include vomiting, which may occur in isolation from nausea. Before the BPAF was revised, pain was only represented as chest pain or pain on micturition, although pain is a principal symptom in all body systems. Therefore 'abdominal pain/distension' was added to the gastrointestinal system. Specifying response of 'yes' or 'no' to the 'bowels open' item was intended to eliminate confusion. 'Constipated stool' was changed to 'hard, dry stool' as a more precise term. The item 'other abnormality' was added to represent changes in bowel habit, altered colour and appearance of stool, and pain on defecation.

Minor changes were made to the urinary section. 'Pain on micturition' was substituted by 'dysuria', which also incorporated difficulty in passing urine or hesitancy, and poor stream for male patients. 'Urgency' was also added to the 'frequency' item, as both are common urinary symptoms. Changes were made to the neuromuscular section. Again pain in this system was absent and therefore 'headache' and 'joint/muscular pain' were added. 'Tingling' was changed to 'paraesthesiae', which includes altered sensations of numbness, 'pins and needles' and tightness. The item 'lethargic' was expanded to include 'mood change', which was thought appropriate to include as it is an important symptom of organic brain disease, metabolic disorders and drug reactions. Similarly 'disorientated' was expanded to include 'confused', which is a common presentation of almost any disorder in elderly people. The item 'contracture/spasticity' was changed to 'contracture/ stiffness', which is easier to understand and may help identify problems with joint movement before it becomes established. Two further items added as a result of expert opinion are 'joint/tissue swelling' and 'rash'.

In addition to decisions to add appropriate signs and symptoms to the BPAF, there were purposeful decisions to exclude others. It was recognized that there were similarities between a medical examination and assessment using the BPAF. The major difference was that the main aim of a medical examination is to produce a diagnosis whereas the main aim of assessment using the BPAF is to identify the presence of new abnormal signs or symptoms. This differentiation helped to exclude some abnormal signs and symptoms on the basis that they were details used to make a diagnosis and were part of a very detailed examination. Examples of these are: abnormal carotid pulse or position of apex beat, abnormal heart sounds, abnormal tendon reflexes.

It was decided to use the technique of auscultation to assess the respiratory system, as it would aid assessment of chest infection and mild heart failure. However, it was decided not to use the techniques of percussion and palpation as these would considerably lengthen the time taken to conduct the assessment. It was suggested that the neurological system be assessed further, including an assessment of muscle power on a scale of 1 to 5. However, this is contrary to the purpose of the BPAF as a means to assess the presence or absence of abnormal signs and symptoms, therefore the suggestion was not incorporated.

Changes in item definition

A number of item definitions were changed as a result of expert opinion. There were too many changes to discuss them all, but a few illustrative examples are given here. Generally the definitions and guidelines for item assessment were expanded to increase comprehensiveness and made more specific to reduce differences in interpretation (see Tables 2.5 and 2.6).

During the consideration of these definitions, it became apparent that some signs and symptoms were connected and could be assessed within the same item on the BPAF, thus incorporating more signs and symptoms without increasing the length of the BPAF, which could easily become unwieldy. An example of this is the assessment of an irregular heart rate, which also involves asking the patient about the presence of palpitations. Another example is that nocturia can be thought of as a type of frequency. Thus in this situation the item definition was revised to encompass all appropriate facets of item assessment.

The layout of the table changed to divide assessment definition and the possible significance of abnormality. This was thought to add

Table 2.5. Item definitions before expert advice

Item on BPAF	Definition
Sputum	Patients may not know the term 'sputum', 'phlegm' may be better. Sputum is a respiratory tract secretion produced with certain conditions. Can be serous (clear, watery or frothy, e.g. in pulmonary oedema), mucoid (clear, grey or white, e.g. in chronic bronchitis/chronic asthma) or purulent (yellow, green or brown, e.g. in pulmonary infection)

Table 2.6. Item definitions after expert advice

Item on BPAF	Assessment definition	Possible significance of abnormality
Sputum	Sputum is a respiratory tract secretion produced with certain abnormal conditions. Amount produced in 24 hours, appearance and duration should be determined. Assessed by patient report and direct observation. Patients may not know the term 'sputum', 'phlegm' may be better. Ideally sputum should be collected and the amount measured, otherwise patients can often give a useful guide to volume in terms of an egg cupful or cupful in 24 hours	Appearance can be serous (clear, watery or frothy, e.g. in pulmonary oedema), mucoid (clear, grey or white, e.g. in chronic bronchitis/ chronic asthma) or purulent (yellow, green or brown, e.g. in pulmonary infection). Haemoptysis is when blood is coughed up. This needs to be differentiated from haematemesis and nasopharyngeal bleeding. Haemoptysis is likely when blood definitely comes up with a cough, is mixed with or streaked in the sputum. Blood from the chest is usually bright red, not brown. Occurs in several conditions, e.g. pulmonary infarction (associated with pleuritic pain and breathless-ness), pneumonia (associated with fever, purulent sputum and signs of consolidation)

clarity to the table, which is intended to be used in conjunction with the BPAF. A complete version of the final copy of the definition table can be found in Appendix 9.

Conclusion

This chapter has described the process taken to examine and develop the BPAF. The information gained from the review of the development of assessment tools in Chapter 1 has been used to guide the strategies selected and the way the process has been presented, in that the report should be detailed to enable a judgement to be made regarding the appropriateness of decisions made.

The work done to refine the BPAF has resulted in a change to its structure. The final version is a 56-item checklist comprised of six sections: respiratory, cardiovascular, temperature, gastrointestinal, urinary and neuromuscular. The remainder of the previous version and the way it is used is still applicable. Overall, the BPAF has not changed greatly and the changes made are intended to improve its performance in its designated purpose. The next chapter reports on the reliability testing of the BPAF.

Chapter 3
Evaluation of the reliability of the Byron Physical Assessment Framework

This chapter reports on the reliability testing of the BPAF and includes a discussion of appropriate approaches to reliability testing, the data collection and analysis methods used, and a report of the findings obtained.

Approach taken

As discussed in Chapter 1, there are three aspects of reliability to assess when testing instruments:

- stability
- equivalence
- internal consistency.

To test the reliability of the BPAF, the only appropriate aspect of reliability to assess is the instrument's equivalence. This was assessed using an inter-rater method whereby two assessors independently assessed the same patient using the BPAF. The assessment of parallel forms reliability as an estimate of the BPAF's equivalence was inappropriate, as no instruments similar to the BPAF were available.

Testing the BPAF's stability by assessing test-retest reliability was also inappropriate. There are several reasons for this. First, the BPAF is not designed to assess a stable trait and therefore it would be impossible to determine whether the assessment was inaccurate or the patient's condition had changed. Second, by reducing the time interval between assessments to minimize the possibility of a change in the patient's condition, the likelihood of memory affecting the patient's responses and the assessors' judgements would be a great deal higher, resulting in falsely high estimates of reliability. Furthermore, a patient's condition can change very quickly and therefore however short the interval between assessments, a change in the patient may still occur.

It is also not appropriate to test the internal consistency of the BPAF. Testing internal consistency involves estimating the extent to which subparts or items of an instrument are all measuring the same attribute. The BPAF does not claim to measure one attribute. While it could be thought to be measuring 'medical stability', this is too flimsy a concept, involving diverse interpretation from 'fit to transfer out of ITU' to 'fit to discharge home'. Even if an acceptable definition was found, it is extremely unlikely that all items of the BPAF would contribute equally to its measurement. Fundamentally, the BPAF was not developed to measure one attribute specifically. It was written to serve a purpose as a checklist to aid systematic assessment. The items on the BPAF are very diverse, e.g. headache and reddening of pressure areas. Therefore internal consistency is not an appropriate aspect of reliability to estimate in the BPAF.

Aims and objectives

This second phase dealt with the second and third aims of the study: 'To test the reliability of the BPAF by examining agreement between assessors' and 'To teach a novice to use the BPAF and examine inter-rater reliability between the novice and an experienced assessor'. To fulfil these aims, the following objectives were set:

- To examine inter-rater reliability between two independent assessors using the BPAF to assess patients being cared for on the NLIU.
- To assess whether this inter-rater reliability is stable over time.
- To examine inter-rater reliability between expert assessors while assessing patients on acute wards.
- To teach two novice assessors how to use the BPAF.
- To assess inter-rater reliability between one expert and one novice assessor.
- To assess reliability as a whole incorporating all the assessments carried out.

Method of investigation

Sample

While it was hoped to look at a sample of 40-50 patients from the NLIU within the data collection period, this was found to be very unrealistic during the early stages of the study because of the slow throughput of patients and the delay in a planned expansion in number of nurse-led beds on the NLIU. Therefore the entire population of the NLIU was assessed at three-weekly intervals.

In addition to this, a sample of at least 25 patients from the acute wards in the same large inner city teaching hospital who had been referred to the NLIU was sought. Due to the size of the available population, both the sample from the NLIU and the sample on the acute wards were the entire population within the convenient time frame.

Site

The site of the study was a NLIU situated in a large inner city teaching hospital. Although some patients were assessed on the acute wards of the same hospital, the assessments were all conducted by NLIU staff as part of the operation of the service provided by the NLIU.

Ethical issues

Approval for the study was sought from the local Research Ethics Committee. Once this was gained, access to approach patients was requested from the NDU leader, and the senior nurses and ward managers of the areas where patients were to be recruited.

All patients who were approached to participate in the study were given a full explanation of the purpose of the study and what would be involved should they agree to participate, i.e. that the assessment would take approximately 15-20 minutes, would entail answering some questions about whether they were experiencing certain symptoms and a brief, non-invasive physical examination. They were assured of confidentiality and of their right to withdraw at any stage during the research without affecting the subsequent care they would receive. Written consent was sought from patients who agreed to participate or from relatives of patients who could not consent themselves. The exclusion of patients who could not consent themselves was considered on ethical grounds, however it was decided to include them on the basis that they would be assessed by the NLIU staff using the assessment framework whether part of the research or not. Therefore it was considered very important to include this patient group when testing the reliability of the framework.

The purpose of the research and the implications of the possible results were explained to each member of the NLIU staff to ensure they did not feel uncomfortable in any way (Polit and Hungler 1987).

Pilot work

Extensive piloting was not thought to be necessary, as the BPAF had been used by NLIU staff for over two years. However, the data collection methods were piloted with five patients on the NLIU to test their feasibility, identify any extraneous factors that may affect the data collected, and ensure that explanations of the study are acceptable and understandable to patients. The pilot study data were used to explore methods of data analysis and to familiarize the researchers with statistical analysis computer software. Few difficulties were experienced, although the need to standardize the calibre of stethoscope used, i.e. Littman ™, was identified.

Preparation for data collection

Prior to its use on the NLIU, the revised BPAF and the definition of items table were circulated to all NLIU staff and presented at a ward meeting to discuss the changes and the reasons why these had been made. There were also informal discussions with permanent staff to address individual enquiries. All members of qualified NLIU staff had participated in an education programme prior to this study conducted by members of the NLIU staff who had completed a post-registration physical assessment module. Written information for staff prepared as part of this education programme can be found in Appendix 1.

All the experienced staff who were involved in assessing patients for the reliability testing were involved as experts in the revision of the tool. As such, it was assumed that they were informed about how to use the revised BPAF to assess a patient.

Aim three of the study was to teach a novice to use the BPAF and examine inter-rater reliability between the novice and experienced assessor. The research assistants working on the NLIU had no experience of using the BPAF. Therefore two teaching seminars were arranged. The first seminar dealt briefly with the way the BPAF was developed and revised, its purpose and how it is used. Each item of the BPAF was discussed in turn, generally following the contents of the definition of items table (see Appendix 9), covering how the item should be assessed, and normal and abnormal findings. The second seminar was a practical session where a consenting patient was assessed using the BPAF and each item was discussed in turn, giving the research assistants the opportunity to go through the assessment of each item. Any items they were uncertain about were addressed further. The greatest concern was assessing altered chest sounds by auscultation and therefore a range of patients on the unit known to have altered chest sounds were asked to allow assessment of their respiration for teaching purposes. This second session continued until the research assistants felt confident they would be able to assess each item on the BPAF.

Data collection process

On the NLIU

Each patient on the NLIU taking part in the study was assessed by the same two assessors, the primary nurse and the researcher. The two assessments were carried out separately, but the second assessment took place as soon after the first as practicable. This minimized the possibility of change in the patient's physical condition but at the same time did not allow each assessor to observe the other. When assessing confused patients or items that are best assessed by direct observation (e.g. colour/consistency of stool, concentrated urine or wound infection) when it was not an appropriate time to observe them, the nurse looking after the patient at the appropriate time or the nursing notes were consulted.

To assess the stability of this inter-rater reliability over time, data collection was conducted in four episodes, with an interval of at least three weeks between them and for statistical purposes these were divided into two periods, the first two episodes being period 1 and the second two episodes being period 2.

On the acute wards

Patients on the acute wards taking part in this study were assessed by either two nurses experienced in using the BPAF (one of the two NLIU assessment nurses and the researcher) or one nurse experienced in using the BPAF and one nurse with minimal experience of using the BPAF but who had some preparation in its use as described earlier (one of the NLIU research assistants and the researcher or one of the assessment nurses). The timing of assessments and the combination of assessors depended on factors related to the operation of the NLIU and were thus beyond the control of this study. Once a patient consented to participate, the data collection procedure was the same as on the NLIU with the exception that the time interval between assessments was more difficult to control due to the pressures of work of the NLIU staff. Thus time intervals between the two assessments tended to be longer than the time intervals between assessments conducted on the NLIU. Forty eight percent of the paired assessments were completed within one hour, 24% were completed within three hours and 28% were completed within five hours.

The researcher did not intervene with any clinical decisions made by the member of the NLIU team unless patient welfare was thought to be jeopardized in some way. Similarly, on the acute wards findings were not communicated to the nursing staff unless any abnormal findings caused concern, e.g. high blood pressure, laboured breathing.

Data analysis techniques

The data obtained were analysed to estimate inter-rater agreement of assessment of BPAF items. The majority of items on the BPAF constitute nominal or dichotomous data, i.e. the sign or symptom is either present or absent. Five of the BPAF items constitute ratio or continuous data, i.e. respiratory rate, heart rate, blood pressure, body temperature and body weight.

Analysis of nominal data

The nominal data of the BPAF was analysed using total percentage agreement and Cohen's Kappa (Cohen 1960), both accepted statistical methods of assessing inter-rater reliability of nominal data (Topf 1986). These methods of analysis of nominal data where the frequency of agreement or disagreement between independent raters for one event or category is assessed, generally use contingency tables to arrange data (see Figure 3.1).

Total percentage agreement is the percentage of times that both raters agree on the occurrence or non-occurrence of an event. The formula used in this study is:

$$\text{Total \% agreement} = \frac{\text{Frequency of agreed occurrence} + \text{Frequency of agreed non-occurrence}}{\text{Total number of assessments}} \times 100.$$

Considering the example in Figure 3.1, where two nurses have independently assessed 100 patients for the presence or absence of an

	Rater 1		
	Occurrence (+)	Non-occurrence (−)	Total
Rater 2 Occurrence (+)	20	15	35
Non-occurrence (−)	15	50	65
Total	35	65	100

Figure 3.1. Hypothetical agreement between two nurses assessing 100 patients for presence or absence of an irregular heart rate. Based on Brennan and Silman (1992).

irregular heart rate, there is a level of 70% agreement between them. However, it is widely accepted that percentage agreement does not discriminate between actual agreement and agreement that arises due to chance. Cohen's Kappa statistic attempts to correct for this by comparing the observed amount of agreement with the expected amount of agreement, which represents agreement due to chance. From the example in Figure 3.1, the observed proportion of agreement (P_o) is the proportion of agreements of the presence (20/100) and absence (50/100) of an irregular heart rate and therefore is 0.70. As both assessors scored 35% of patients as having an irregular heart rate, then by chance alone the proportion that would be assessed as present by both assessors is 35/100 × 35/100 = 0.12. Similarly the expected chance proportion of agreed assessment of absence is 65/100 × 65/100 = 0.42 giving a total expected agreement (P_e) of 0.54. The Kappa statistic (κ) represents the extra amount of agreement observed after taking into account chance ($P_o - P_e$) divided by the maximum amount of such agreement that could theoretically occur ($1 - P_e$). Therefore the computational formula used in this study is:

$$\kappa = \frac{(P_o - P_e)}{(1 - P_e)} \qquad \text{(Brennan and Silman 1992).}$$

For the data in Figure 3.1:

$$\kappa = \frac{(0.70 - 0.54)}{(1 - 0.54)} = 0.34$$

A contingency table was complete for each of the nominal data items of the BPAF and percentage agreement, expected agreement and κ computed for the following groups of data:

- first period of assessments completed on the NLIU patients
- second period of assessments completed on the NLIU patients
- total assessments completed on the NLIU
- novice/experienced assessors' assessments
- experienced assessors' assessments completed on the acute wards
- total assessments completed during whole study.

For each group of data a contingency table was completed combining the frequencies of agreement and disagreement for every item to give a total percentage agreement and κ score for the BPAF in each of the above circumstances.

What is good agreement?

Waltz et al. (1991) consider that the values of percentage agreement and κ as an acceptable level of inter-rater agreement varies from situation to situation. However, they cite 'safe guidelines' for acceptable levels as being 80% or above for percentage agreement and 0.25 or above for κ. Both Landis and Koch (1977) and Altman (1991) have suggested arbitrary interpretation of agreement for different values of κ and these can be found in Table 3.1. The range of κ is –1, indicating perfect disagreement to +1 indicating perfect agreement.

Table 3.1. Comparison of Landis and Koch's and Altman's interpretation of agreement for different values of κ

Landis and Koch (1977)		Altman (1991)	
κ statistic	Strength of agreement	κ statistic	Strength of agreement
0.00	poor		
0.01–0.20	slight	< 0.20	poor
0.21–0.40	fair	0.21–0.40	fair
0.41–0.60	moderate	0.41–0.60	moderate
0.61–0.80	substantial	0.61–0.80	good
0.81–1.00	almost perfect	0.81–1.00	very good

These interpretations of agreement are very similar and Altman's version was chosen for use in this study because there seemed little value in distinguishing 0.00 as poor and 0.01 as slight, as interpreted by Landis and Koch (1977). The only report of acceptable percentage agreement found was that of Waltz et al.

Analysis of ratio data

The use of Pearson's correlation coefficient as a method to assess variation in raters' observations recorded on a continuous scale is considered to be inappropriate by Bland and Altman (1986) as it assesses the association between the raters but does not identify consistent bias such as one rater constantly recording twice the value of the other.

Bland and Altman (1986) consider that a more meaningful representation of the level of variability is to plot the difference between each of the assessors recordings against the corresponding mean of those recordings. Therefore a scatter plot was constructed, using Minitab™ statistical package, for each of the groups of data outlined above. The standard deviation of the difference between the raters' scores was calculated to examine inter-rater reliability. This gives an indication of the variability of the scores obtained. The formula used to calculate standard deviation (s) is:

$$s = \sqrt{\frac{(x_1 - \bar{x})^2 + \ldots + (x_n - \bar{x})^2}{n - 1}}$$

To assess the level of agreement between assessors more accurately, the 95% tolerance interval within which 95% of differences between assessors would lie was calculated. To do this, the range within which most of their disagreements occurred was calculated, based on the mean difference between assessors ($\bar{d}$) and the standard deviation (see above) of these differences(s_{diff}), using the following formula:

Range of disagreement between assessors $= \bar{d} \pm t_{n-1} s_{\text{diff}}$
where t_{n-1} is the appropriate probability point of the t distribution of n–1 degrees of freedom for 95%.
For larger samples ($n > 50$) the 95% range $= \bar{d} \pm 2s_{\text{diff}}$

For the tolerance interval the larger value of this range is subtracted from the smaller value to find the maximum extent of the range and divided by 2. This 95% tolerance interval represents the value within which the differences between the assessors would lie 95% of the time.

To measure existing bias between assessors and an indication of the strength of any possible bias, a 95% confidence interval for was calculated using the standard error of the mean difference. Formula used is:

Confidence interval for $\bar{d} = \bar{d} \pm t_{n-1}\text{SE}$ where $\text{SE} = \dfrac{s_{\text{diff}}}{\sqrt{n}}$

If zero lies outside this confidence interval then it can be concluded that bias exists between assessors (Brennan and Silman 1992).

Findings

Sixty eight patients were assessed in total. Of these, 21 were assessed during the first two episodes of assessments conducted on the NLIU patients and 22 were assessed during the second two episodes. Seventeen patients were assessed by one novice assessor and one experienced assessor on the acute wards, and eight patients were assessed by two experienced assessors as part of the screening procedure on the acute wards.

The findings will be presented in line with the objectives of this phase of the study. Findings are reported in full with examples of raw data in Harris (1995). Where signs and symptoms were not assessed as present by either of the two assessors in any of the patient assessments, the κ statistic cannot be computed and no inference can be made about inter-rater agreement for those items.

Objective 1. To examine inter-rater reliability between two independent assessors using the BPAF to assess patients being cared for on the NLIU

To fulfil this objective, data from the total number (n = 43) of NLIU assessments will be presented.

Nominal data

The percentage agreement of all nominal items of the BPAF ranged from 74% to 100%, with only two items below the safe acceptable levels (80%) cited by Waltz et al. (1991). Moreover 41/51 of these nominal items had a percentage agreement of over 90%.

The k statistic of all nominal items of the BPAF ranged from 0.00 to 1.00. The numbers of items achieving each strength of agreement as interpreted by Altman (1991) are presented in Table 3.2.

Table 3.2. Number of nominal items of the total NLIU assessments achieving each strength of agreement specified by Altman

Strength of agreement of κ statistic (Altman 1991)		No. of items achieving strength of agreement
No κ obtained		3
< 0.20	(poor)	3
0.21–0.40	(fair)	4
0.41–0.60	(moderate)	5
0.61–0.80	(good)	17
0.81–1.00	(very good)	19

Table 3.3 shows items with unacceptable % agreement and poor or fair κ agreement.

Table 3.3. Nominal items with low level of agreement in the total NLIU assessments

Items failing to achieve acceptable % agreement scores of 80% (Waltz et al. 1991)	Items achieving only poor (< 0.20) or fair (0.21–0.40) agreement for κ statistic (Altman 1991)
• dry mouth • joint/muscular pain	• chest pain • reduced tissue turgor • dry mouth • hard, dry stool • concentrated urine • paraesthesiae • rash

The total percentage agreement score and κ statistic for all items combined giving one score for this group of assessments are 93% and 0.79 respectively.

Ratio data

Figure 3.2 shows the scatter plots constructed for each of the ratio data items. Each of these scatter plots shows that there is considerable range of disagreement in the assessments. For example, Figure 3.2a shows discrepancies of up to 11 breaths/minute in respiratory rate, Figure 3.2b shows discrepancies of up to 34 beats/minute in heart rate and Figure 3.2d shows discrepancies of up to 50 mmHg in systolic blood pressure. To assess the level of agreement between assessors more accurately, the

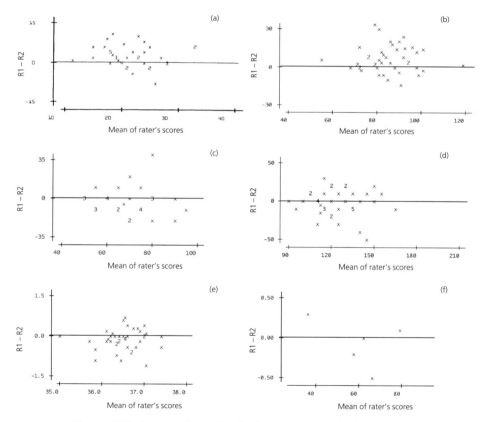

Figure 3.2. Scatter plots of ratio data of the total number of assessments conducted on the NLIU patients (*n = 43), where the difference between raters' scores (R1 - R2) is plotted against the mean of the raters' scores. (a) Respiratory rate (breaths/min); (b) heart rate (beats/min); (c) diastolic BP (mmHg); (d) systolic BP (mmHg); (e) temperature (°C); (f) weight (kg). '+' represents 9 or more points.*

standard deviation of the differences between assessors' scores, the range within which most disagreements occurred and the confidence level for the mean difference between assessors ($\bar{d}$) are presented in Table 3.4.

Table 3.4. Data to assess the level of agreement for ratio data between assessors in the total number of NLIU assessments

Item on BPAF	Standard deviation of the difference between assessors scores	95% tolerance interval of the difference between the two assessors	95% confidence interval for $\bar{d}$
Respiratory rate	3.76	7.59	1.26 to 3.58
Diastolic BP	10.72	21.65	−5.60 to 1.08
Systolic BP	16.61	33.54	−8.03 to 2.32
Heart rate	10.18	26.94	3.26 to 9.53
Temperature	0.39	0.78	−0.26 to −0.01
Weight	0.31	0.88	−0.44 to 0.32

To illustrate the inferences made from the data, it can be seen from Table 3.4 that in the case of respiratory rate, on average the difference between the two assessors scores deviates by 3.76 breaths/min from the mean difference between the two assessors scores. The 95% tolerance interval for respiratory rate shows that 95% of the time the assessors' scores would be within 7.59 breaths. Since zero is not included in the 95% confidence interval for $\bar{d}$, there is evidence that there is bias between the two assessors with rater 1 consistently assessing respiratory rate higher than rater 2. All these physical signs show a fairly high level of variability and bias is also found in heart rate recording with rater 1 assessing higher than rater 2.

Objective 2. To assess whether this inter-rater reliability is stable over time

To fulfil this objective, data from the first period of assessments conducted on the NLIU will be compared with the second period of assessments conducted on the NLIU.

Nominal data

The percentage agreement of all nominal items ranged from 67% to 100% for the first two episodes to 68% to 100% for the second two episodes. Four items failed to attain acceptable levels (80%) in the first compared with only one item of the second period of assessments. In the first period of assessments, 39/51 of items achieved an agreement level of 90%, whereas 45/51 achieved this level in the second period.

The κ statistic of all nominal items on the BPAF ranged from 0.00 to 1.00 in both episodes of assessments. The number of items achieving each strength of agreement as specified by Altman are presented in Table 3.5. Table 3.6 shows items with unacceptable percentage agreement and poor or fair κ agreement.

Table 3.5. A comparison of number of nominal items of each period of NLIU assessments achieving each strength of agreement

Strength of agreement of κ statistic (Altman 1991)	No. of items achieving strength of agreement First two episodes of assessments	No. of items achieving strength of agreement Second two episodes of assessments
No κ obtained	5	8
< 0.20 (poor)	3	7
0.21–0.40 (fair)	5	2
0.41–0.60 (moderate)	5	2
0.61–0.80 (good)	14	10
0.81–1.00 (very good)	19	22

Table 3.6. A comparison of the nominal items with low level of agreement in each of the two periods of NLIU assessments

Items failing to achieve acceptable % agreement scores of 80% (Waltz et al. 1991)		Items achieving only poor (< 0.20) or fair (0.21–0.40) agreement for κ statistic (Altman 1991)	
Period 1	Period 2	Period 1	Period 2
• pale skin	• dry mouth	• chest pain	• reduced tissue turgor
• reduced tissue turgor		• hard/dry stool	• coated mouth
• poor appetite		• concentrated urine	• hard, dry stool
• joint/muscular pain		• reduced tissue turgor	• dysuria
		• dry mouth	• visual disturbance
		• paraesthesiae	• joint/tissue swelling
		• joint/muscular pain	• rash
		• rash	• dry mouth
			• paraesthesiae

The percentage agreement and κ statistic for total agreements and disagreements for every item in these groups of data are 93% and 0.76 for the first two episodes of assessments and 94% and 0.83 for the second two episodes of assessments.

Ratio data

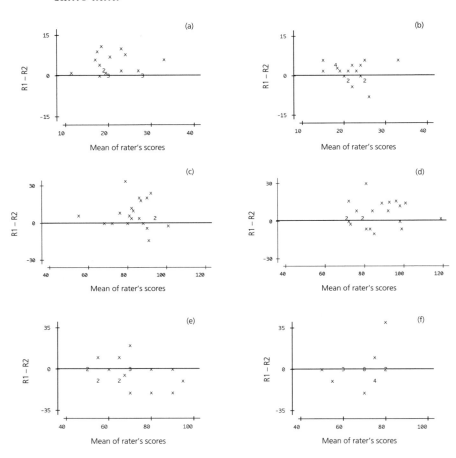

Figure 3.3. Scatter plots of ratio data of period 1 (left) and period 2 (right) of assessments conducted on the NLIU patients (n = 21 and 22 respectively), where the difference between raters' scores (R1 - R2) is plotted against the mean of the raters' score. (a) Respiratory rate (breaths/min); (b) respiratory rate (breaths/min); (c) heart rate (beats/min); (d) heart rate (beats/min); (e) diastolic BP (mmHg); (f) diastolic BP (mmHg); (g) systolic BP (mmHg); (h) systolic BP (mmHg); (i) temperature (°C); (j) temperature (°C).

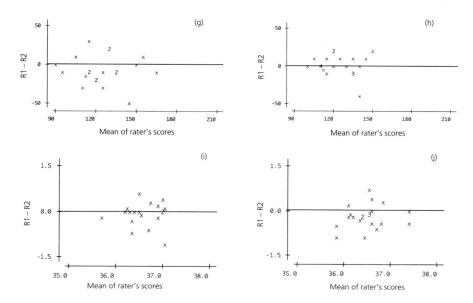

Figure 3.3. (contd).

Figure 3.3 shows the scatter plots constructed for each of the ratio items in the first two episodes and second two episodes of assessments. The two scatter plots for each item are arranged alongside each other to allow easy comparison. Again a considerable range of disagreement between assessors is presented. There is no obvious pattern of this disagreement between each set of episodes of assessments for all items. However, a tendency for rater 1 to assess respiratory rate and heart rate higher than rater 2 can be seen in both scatter plots, as a majority of the graph points occur above the zero line.

The standard deviation of the differences between assessors' scores (see Table 3.7) show similarity between the first two and second two episodes of assessments, with the exception of systolic BP, where the later assessments show a marked decrease in score differences. Moreover, with the exception of diastolic BP, the later assessments of items show greater agreement between assessors.

The tolerance intervals (see Table 3.7) show that with the exception of diastolic BP, there is lower variability between assessors in period 2 of assessments. The 95% confidence level for $\bar{d}$ shows that bias exists between raters in earlier assessments in respiratory rate and heart rate recordings, confirming the data shown in the scatter plots. In later

Table 3.7. Data to compare the level of agreement between assessors in period 1 and period 2 of NLIU assessments

Item on BPAF	Standard deviation of the difference between assessors' scores		95% tolerance interval for the difference between assessors' scores		95% confidence interval for $\bar{d}$	
	Period 1	Period 2	Period 1	Period 2	Period 1	Period 2
Respiratory rate	3.75	3.62	7.82	7.53	1.72 to 7.68	−0.11 to 3.11
Diastolic BP	10.37	11.09	21.71	23.06	−8.60 to 1.10	−5.83 to 4.01
Systolic BP	19.02	13.27	39.81	27.59	−16.15 to 1.65	−4.75 to 7.02
Heart rate	10.92	9.59	22.79	19.94	2.36 to 12.31	1.25 to 9.75
Temperature	0.39	0.38	0.83	0.79	−0.27 to 0.11	−0.35 to −0.01
Weight	No data	0.31	No data	0.85	No data	−0.44 to 0.32

assessments, bias between raters still exists for heart rate, although it is slightly reduced. Assessments of respiratory rate no longer show bias, but temperature recordings show that there is bias, with rater 1 consistently rating temperature as lower than rater 2.

Objective 3. To examine inter-rater reliability between experienced assessors while screening patients on acute wards

Nominal data

The percentage agreement of the nominal items ranged from 38% to 100%, with 14 items failing to achieve the safe acceptable level (80%); 23/51 items had a percentage agreement of over 90%.

Table 3.8. Number of nominal items of the assessments by two experienced assessors achieving each strength of agreement specified by Altman (1991)

Strength of agreement of κ statistic (Altman 1991)	No. of items achieving strength of agreement
No κ obtained	6
< 0.20 (poor)	4
0.21–0.40 (fair)	7
0.41–0.60 (moderate)	8
0.61–0.80 (good)	9
0.81–1.00 (very good)	17

The κ statistic of all nominal items ranged from -0.25 to 1.00. The number of items achieving each strength of agreement as interpreted by Altman (1991) are presented in Table 3.8. Table 3.9 shows items with unacceptable percentage agreement and poor or fair κ agreement.

The percentage agreement and κ statistic for the total number of agreements and disagreements for every item in this group of data are 88% and 0.72 respectively.

Table 3.9. Nominal items with low level of agreement in assessments by two experienced assessors on acute wards

Items failing to achieve acceptable percentage agreement scores of 80% (Waltz et al. 1991)		Items achieving only poor (< 0.20) or fair (0.21–0.40) agreement for κ statistic (Altman 1991)	
• resp: other abnormality	• cough	• resp: other abnormality	• pale skin
• reddening of pressure areas	• dizziness	• skin: cool/ clammy	• coated mouth
• lethargic/mood change	• pale skin	• reduced tissue turgor	• dysuria
• disorientated/ confused	• coated mouth	• visual disturbance	• contracture/ stiffness
• joint/muscular swelling	• skin: cool/ clammy	• lethargic/mood change	
• joint/tissue swelling	• visual disturbance	• disorientated/ confused	
• reduced tissue turgor	• contracture/ stiffness	• reddening of pressure areas	

Ratio data

Figure 3.4 shows the scatter plots for each of the ratio items. Again these scatter plots display the extent of disagreement between assessors. The small number of assessments ($n = 8$) enhances this dispersion, although a pattern of disagreement is not obvious, with the exception of diastolic BP where the recordings of rater 1 are always higher or equal to rater 2. This visual bias in the recording of diastolic BP is confirmed by the 95% confidence interval of the mean difference between assessors (see Table 3.10) which statistically supports this bias. The standard deviation of the differences between scores of two experienced assessors screening a patient are presented in Table 3.10 and show the highest variability for respiratory rate, heart rate and temperature recording in this study.

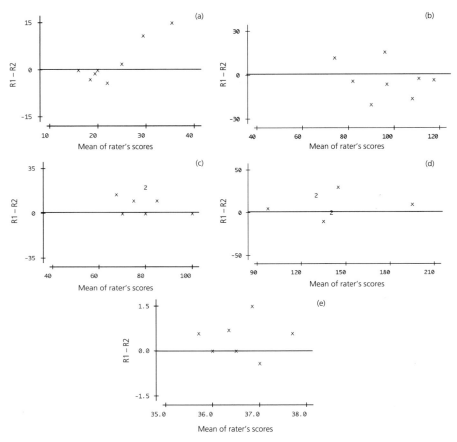

Figure 3.4. Scatter plots of ratio data of the assessments by two experienced assessors conducted on the acute wards ($n = 8$) where the difference between raters' scores (R1 - R2) is plotted against the mean of the raters' scores. (a) Respiratory rate (breaths/min); (b) heart rate (beats/min); (c) diastolic BP (mmHg); (d) systolic BP (mmHg); (e) temperature (°C).

Table 3.10. Data to assess the level of agreement for ratio data between two experienced assessors

Item on BPAF	Standard deviation of the difference between assessors scores	95% tolerance interval for the difference between assessors scores	95% confidence interval for $\bar{d}$
Respiratory rate	6.82	16.14	−3.21 to 8.21
Diastolic BP	8.15	19.27	2.57 to 16.19
Systolic BP	13.21	31.25	−1.67 to 20.42
Heart rate	12.28	29.03	−13.14 to 7.39
Temperature	0.62	1.53	−0.15 to 1.01
Weight	No data	No data	No data

Objective 5. To assess inter-rater reliability between one experienced and one novice assessor after the novice has received some teaching about the BPAF

Nominal data

The percentage agreement of nominal items ranged from 65% to 100% with 11 items failing to achieve the safe acceptable level (80%); 27/51 items had a percentage agreement of over 90%.

The κ statistic ranged from –0.06 to 1.00. The strength of agreement achieved by each item is presented in Table 3.11. Table 3.12 shows items with unacceptable percentage agreement and poor or fair κ agreement.

Table 3.11. Number of nominal items of the assessments by one novice and one experienced assessor achieving each strength of agreement specified by Altman (1991)

Strength of agreement of κ statistic (Altman 1991)	No. of items achieving strength of agreement
No κ obtained	5
< 0.20 (poor)	8
0.21–0.40 (fair)	7
0.41–0.60 (moderate)	7
0.61–0.80 (good)	10
0.81–1.00 (very good)	14

Table 3.12. Nominal items with low level of agreement in assessments by one novice and one experienced assessor

Items failing to achieve acceptable percentage agreement scores of 80% (Waltz et al. 1991)		Items achieving only poor (< 0.20) or fair (0.21–0.40) agreement for κ statistic (Altman 1991)	
• irregular heart rate	• cough	• pitting oedema	• pale skin
• special diet/ feeding	• pale skin	• skin: cool/ clammy	• reduced tissue turgor
• reduced tissue turgor	• contracture/ stiffness	• rash	• cyanosis - peripheral
• pitting oedema	• dry mouth	• incontinent	• poor appetite
• poor appetite		• frequency/urgency	• added sounds
• frequency/ urgency		• odour	• irregular heart rate
• paraesthesiae		• paraesthesiae	• calf pain/ swelling
		• dry mouth	

The percentage agreement and κ statistic for the total number of agreements and disagreements for every item in this group of data are 89% and 0.62 respectively.

Ratio data

The scatter plots for each item are shown in Figure 3.5. The disagreement displayed does appear less marked than in other groups of assessments. The standard deviations of the difference in assessors' scores

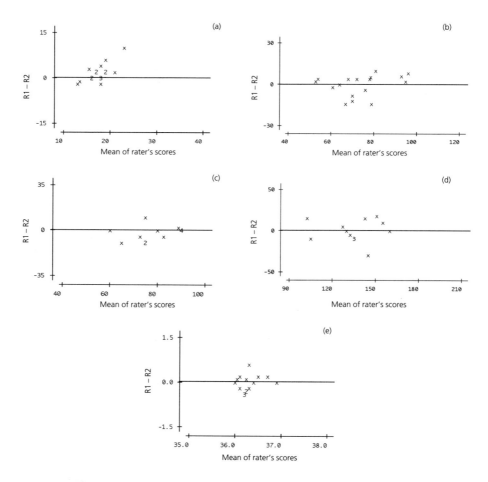

Figure 3.5. Scatter plots of ratio data of the assessments by one novice assessor and one experienced assessor ($n = 17$) where the difference between raters' scores (R1 - R2) is plotted against the mean of the raters' scores. (a) Respiratory rate (breaths/min); (b) heart rate (beats/min); (c) diastolic BP (mmHg); (d) systolic BP (mmHg); (e) temperature (°C).

(see Table 3.13) confirms this decreased variability, as they are the lowest standard deviations in the study for all items except systolic BP. Correspondingly, the 95% tolerance intervals are the lowest in the study for all items except systolic BP, thus indicating a higher agreement between assessors.

The 95% confidence interval for $\bar{d}$ shows that bias exists between assessors in respiratory rate assessment, with the experienced assessors tending to report a higher rate than the novice assessors.

Table 3.13. Data to assess the level of agreement for ratio data between one novice and one experienced assessor

Item on BPAF	Standard deviation of the difference between assessors scores	95% tolerance interval for the difference between assessors scores	95% confidence interval for $\bar{d}$
Respiratory rate	3.00	6.36	0.11 to 3.19
Diastolic BP	5.73	12.48	−5.62 to 1.31
Systolic BP	13.58	29.59	−9.13 to 7.28
Heart rate	7.56	16.04	−4.18 to 3.60
Temperature	0.28	0.60	−0.20 to 0.10
Weight	No data	No data	No data

Objective 6. To assess reliability of the BPAF as a whole incorporating all the assessments carried out

The findings presented in the section on the total number of assessments have been computed from the raw data and as such can be seen as overall findings for the reliability of the BPAF.

Nominal data

The percentage agreement of nominal items ranged from 72% to 100% with three failing to attain a safe acceptable level of 80% (Waltz et al. 1991); 35/51 had a percentage agreement of ≥ 90%.

The κ statistic ranged from 0.20 to 1.00. The strength of agreement achieved by each item is presented in Table 3.14. Table 3.15 shows items with unacceptable percentage agreement and poor or fair κ agreement.

These results show that a larger proportion of items reached a moderate or higher level of agreement than in the other groups of assessments.

The percentage agreement and κ statistic for the total number of agreements and disagreements for every item, giving one overall score for all the assessments completed in the study, are 92% and 0.75 respectively.

Table 3.14. Number of nominal items of the total number of assessments in the study achieving each strength of agreement specified by Altman (1991)

Strength of agreement of κ statistic (Altman 1991)	No. of items achieving strength of agreement
No κ obtained	2
< 0.20 (poor)	1
0.21–0.40 (fair)	5
0.41–0.60 (moderate)	10
0.61–0.80 (good)	16
0.81–1.00 (very good)	17

Table 3.15. Nominal items with low level of agreement in the total number of assessments in the study

Items failing to achieve acceptable % agreement scores of 80% (Waltz et al. 1991)	Items achieving only poor (< 0.20) or fair (0.21–0.40) agreement for κ statistic (Altman 1991)
• pale skin • reduced tissue turgor • dry mouth	• cyanosis - peripheral • pale skin • dry mouth • paraesthesiae • rash • reduced tissue turgor

Ratio data

Figure 3.6 shows the scatter plots for the ratio items of the total number of assessments conducted in the study. In each of these scatter plots, the points appear to be evenly, although fairly widely, dispersed around the zero line, with the exception of respiratory rate, where rater 1 tends to record the rate as higher than rater 2. The 95% confidence interval for $\bar{d}$ presented in Table 3.16 shows that bias exists between raters for both respiratory rate and heart rate recording.

Table 3.16. Data to assess the level of agreement for ratio data between all groups of assessors

Item on BPAF	Standard deviation of the difference between assessors scores	95% tolerance interval for the difference between assessors scores	95% confidence interval for $\bar{d}$
Respiratory rate	4.00	8.01	1.27 to 3.20
Diastolic BP	10.29	20.59	−3.36 to 1.83
Systolic BP	15.94	31.88	−4.92 to 3.11
Heart rate	10.41	20.81	1.11 to 6.16
Temperature	0.43	0.85	−0.16 to 0.05
Weight	No data	No data	No data

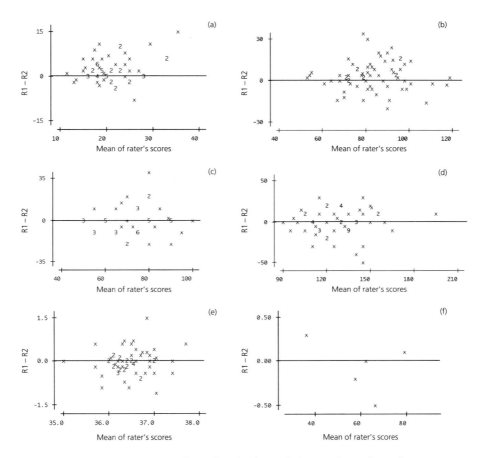

Figure 3.6. Scatter plots of ratio data of the total number of assessments conducted in the study (*n* = 68) where the difference between raters' scores (R1 - R2) is plotted against the mean of the raters' scores. (a) Respiratory rate (breaths/min); (b) heart rate (beats/min); (c) diastolic BP (mmHg); (d) systolic BP (mmHg); (e) temperature (°C); (f) weight (kg). '+' represents 9 or more points.

The implication of all these scores for the inter-rater reliability of the BPAF will be discussed in Chapter 5.

Summary

The findings from the evaluation of the inter-rater reliability of the BPAF are variable, with the agreement between assessors for some nominal items being higher than others (see Table 3.17).

Disagreement between assessors for nominal data was higher among experienced assessors screening patients (highest level of unacceptable

Table 3.17. Nominal items with consistently high and low agreement between assessors

Nominal items with consistent high agreement between assessors ($\kappa \geq 0.61$ in all groups)		Nominal items with frequent poor or fair agreement between assessors ($\kappa \leq 0.40$ in 2 or more groups)	
• laboured/ breathless	• sputum	• cyanosis - peripheral	• pale skin
• weak pulse	• skin: hot	• skin: cool/ clammy	• reduced tissue turgor
• nausea/ vomiting	• dysphagia	• dry mouth	• coated mouth
• bowels open	• loose stool	• hard, dry stool	• dysuria
• faecal incontinence	• catheterized	• visual disturbance	• paraesthesiae
• slurred speech/ dysarthric	• dysphasic	• rash	
• limb: weakness/ flaccid	• skin ulceration		
• other abnormality (bowel)	• purulent wound		

percentage agreement scores) and the assessments conducted by one novice assessor and one experienced assessor (highest level of unacceptable κ correlations). This is illustrated in Table 3.18, where the total percentage agreement and κ statistic for the agreement and disagreement of every item combined are presented.

Table 3.18. The total percentage agreement and κ for the agreement and disagreement of every item combined for each of the groups of data

Group of assessments		Percentage agreement	κ statistic
Objective 1	- Total NLIU assessments	93	0.79
Objective 2	- Episodes 1 & 2, NLIU	93	0.76
	- Episodes 3 & 4, NLIU	94	0.83
Objective 3	- Two experienced assessors	88	0.72
Objective 5	- Novice and experienced assessors	89	0.62
Objective 6	- Total of all assessments in study	92	0.75

The agreement between assessors for the ratio data was varied, with the highest agreement among the novice and experienced assessors and the lowest among the experienced assessors screening patients on acute wards. The standard deviation of the difference in assessors' scores and the 95% tolerance interval show a high degree of variability at times and the implications of these scores for the reliability of the BPAF will be discussed in Chapter 5. The confidence intervals for the mean of the differences in assessors' scores show that bias in recording the ratio data has occurred, particularly in respiratory rate and heart rate recording.

Chapter 4
Evaluation of the validity of the Byron Physical Assessment Framework

This chapter reports on the evaluation of the validity testing of the BPAF, and includes discussion of appropriate approaches to validity testing of the BPAF, the data collected and a report of the findings.

Approach taken

As discussed in Chapter 1, there are four types of validity to assess when testing instruments: face validity, content validity, criterion-related validity and construct validity. For the BPAF, the only type that is appropriate is content validity. This was assessed by careful examination of accepted medical texts concerning physical assessment and consultation with experts in physical assessment, assessment tool development and experienced users of the BPAF.

Testing the face validity of the BPAF was thought not to be possible due to the nature of the client group, who are frail and elderly. It was thought they would have difficulty in making a judgement about the applicability of the tool, which has a large technical component, and that it may cause distress.

Testing the criterion-related validity of the BPAF was not possible due to the absence of another reliable and valid criterion with which to compare the assessments made using the BPAF. In addition, the BPAF addresses such a diverse area in terms of a patient's physical condition, encompassing assessment of a broad range of physiological indicators that have a very complex inter-relationship. Moreover, the significance of these indicators collectively for the patient's physical condition as a whole is intricate and fraught with multiple influences. As such, a meaningful criterion against which to correlate the findings of the BPAF was not identified.

For similar reasons testing the construct validity, which is essentially concerned with the extent to which an instrument actually measures the theoretical construct that it is designed to measure, was thought to be unfeasible. The BPAF was not developed to measure a specific theoretical construct but rather as a clinical tool to aid systematic assessment. As discussed briefly in Chapter 2, there has been some conjecture about whether there is one broad attribute that the BPAF addresses, but no tangible concept has emerged. However, in their description of validity, Carmines and Zeller (1979) emphasize that it is the validity of the instrument in relation to its purpose that should be tested, not the instrument itself. Similarly, Waltz et al. (1991) consider that one aspect of construct validation is to establish support for the instrument's ability to fulfil the purpose for which it is being used. Therefore the utilization of the BPAF in relation to its purpose was assessed by examining completed assessments and examining the outcome in terms of nurses' actions in light of new abnormal findings.

Aims and objectives

The purpose of this third phase was to fulfil the fourth aim of the study: 'To examine patient assessment documentation retrospectively for evidence of action taken as a result of using the BPAF as an indication of the BPAF's validity'. In addition, there will be some discussion about the assessment of content validity of the BPAF through the work conducted when refining the instrument, which was reported in Chapter 2. Therefore the following objectives were set:

- To examine the process used to refine the BPAF to establish whether content validity is supported.
- To examine completed BPAFs retrospectively to assess how consistently they are completed.
- To examine patient documentation retrospectively for evidence of action taken by nurses as a result of the detection of a new abnormality using the BPAF to assess utilization of the BPAF.

Objective 1. To examine the process used to refine the BPAF to establish whether content validity is supported

Two methodologies were used to refine the BPAF, extensive literature review and expert opinion. Both strategies are commonly used to assess content validity. In describing the process of establishing an instrument's content validity, Carmines and Zeller (1979) suggested that a thorough literature review be conducted to elicit the full scope of content. Waltz et al. (1991) identified the use of 'content specialists' to examine the representativeness of the items within the instrument to measure the content domain of interest as determined by the instrument's specifications for use.

The strategy used to review the literature was selected to gain a comprehensive view of the possible content of the BPAF. This strategy involved selection of accepted medical texts on physical assessment, as this was the content domain of the BPAF. These texts were selected on the advice of a lecturer responsible for the post-registration degree course module on physical assessment. The large amount of possible BPAF content yielded by this review (shown in Figure 2.2 and Appendices 4 to 7), was then used by experts in their consideration of the BPAF's comprehensiveness, clarity and relevance to its intended purpose. These experts were selected on the basis of their knowledge of physical assessment. Some changes were made to the BPAF through the combination of the literature review and discussion among experts, and the revised version was considered to represent a more comprehensive physical assessment of the NLIU's client group.

However, there are no objective methods to assess the adequacy of content coverage of an instrument (Polit and Hungler 1987). Nunnally (1978) considers that 'inevitably content validity rests mainly on appeals to reason regarding the adequacy with which important content has been sampled and on the adequacy with which the content has been cast in the form of test items'. Therefore a judgement of an instrument's content validity rests on the degree of satisfaction in the rigour of procedures used to determine the content, e.g. how the literature to review was selected, how the experts were selected, how consensus of opinion was reached.

Objective 2. To retrospectively examine completed BPAFs to assess how consistently they are completed

The BPAF was designed to be used daily with each patient. To evaluate its effectiveness the frequency with which it was used was also thought to be important.

Method

A sample of 20 sets of notes of patients who had already consented to the study was sought. Sampling took place two months after the use of the revised BPAF had commenced to ensure that staff were accustomed to using the new version. As patients were discharged from the NLIU their notes were examined. At the end of the data collection period, notes of patients who were still inpatients on the NLIU were selected to increase the sample to 20. To gain a sample of 20, every consenting inpatient's notes were selected. Therefore the entire population within the timescale was selected.

For each set of notes, the BPAF's were retrieved and examined to assess the extent to which they were completed. Each day on the BPAF was judged as having been 'completed' where all items were assessed, 'partially completed' where not all the items were assessed or 'not completed' where none of the items was assessed. In some cases, some of the BPAFs were not found and these were classified as 'lost'. The number of 'completed', 'partially completed', 'not completed' and 'lost' BPAFs for each set of notes individually and the 20 sets of notes collectively were added up and percentages of each category computed.

The same exercise was completed for the data collected for the preliminary investigation of the utilization of the BPAF reported in Chapter 2. These data were randomly selected from the notes of patients treated in the first 18 months of the nurse-led service when the first two versions of the BPAF were in use. This allows comparison of the use of previous versions of the BPAF with that of the refined version

Findings

It can be seen from the findings presented in Table 4.1 that there were differences between the previous versions and the revised version of the BPAF in the proportion of completed assessments and those not completed at all. A much higher proportion of earlier assessments were fully completed (53%) compared to recent assessments (32%), a trend that was reversed for assessments that were not completed at all (18% of earlier assessments versus 37% of recent assessments).

Table 4.1. Comparison of the degree of completeness of assessment using the BPAF between earlier assessments using previous versions of the BPAF and recent assessments using the revised version of the BPAF

Category	Range of frequency of each category within the 20 sets of notes (%)		Total frequency of each category for the 20 sets of notes (%)	
	Revised BPAF - June/July 1995	Previous versions of BPAF - Feb 1993 to Sept 1994	Revised BPAF - June/July 1995	Previous versions of BPAF - Feb 1993 to Sept 1994
Completed	4–55	0–93	32	53
Partially completed	0–39	0–74	20	18
Not completed	10–57	6–38	37	18
Lost	0–71	0–41	11	11

The proportions of partially completed assessments and lost assessments were very similar. Of the partially completed assessments, many had just one or two items not assessed. Assessing chest sounds was frequently omitted in both earlier and recent assessments and BP was frequently omitted in the recent assessments. Unlike the earlier assessments, some of the recent assessments were virtually uncompleted with just respiratory rate, heart rate, temperature, blood pressure and whether bowels have been opened having been assessed.

Objective 3. To retrospectively examine patient documentation for evidence of action taken by nurses as a result of the detection of a new abnormality using the BPAF to assess utilization of the BPAF

To assess the extent the instrument fulfils the purpose for which it is being used, patient documentation was examined retrospectively for evidence of action taken by nursing staff as a result of the detection of a new abnormality.

Method

A sample of 100 new abnormalities assessed by a nurse using the BPAF were selected from the same 20 sets of patient casenotes selected for the data collection for objective 2 (see above for sampling technique). Using the same method used for the preliminary investigation of the utilization of the BPAF described in Chapter 2, five consecutive new abnormalities assessed using the BPAF were selected. The action taken as a result of each abnormality was then found by examining the medical notes, nursing notes and the unit doctor's communication book. The action taken in response to assessment of a new abnormal sign or symptom was assigned to three categories:

- no documentation/no action taken
- findings documented/action taken
- referral made to medical or therapy staff.

In some cases, action taken was assigned to more than one category.

Findings

Of the 100 new abnormalities assessed, 17% were referred for medical input: 14% were referred to the unit doctor, 0% were referred back to the referring team and 5% were seen by an on-call SHO for urgent medical input. Some patients were referred for more than one type of medical input at the same time. Of the 14 referrals to the unit doctor,

11 required medical investigation, e.g. blood tests, ECGs and X-rays, and/or treatment, e.g. antibiotics, analgesia and diuretics. Of all new abnormalities, 25% were documented by nursing staff either in medical or nursing notes, and in some cases action was taken to investigate, e.g. blood samples, urine samples or ECG. Overall, 41% of new abnormalities assessed via the revised BPAF were acted on in some way by the nursing staff.

These findings were compared with the earlier assessments using the previous versions of the BPAF, which were reported in Chapter 2 as the 'preliminary investigation of the utilisation of the BPAF', and are presented in Table 4.2.

When comparing the two sets of findings, the proportion of referrals for medical input was lower in recent assessments (17% versus 37%). None of the new abnormalities found in the recent assessments resulted in referring the patient back to their referring medical team, compared with 7% in earlier assessments. Of the referrals for medical input resulting from recent assessments, 14/17 were referred to the unit doctor compared to 31/37 of those resulting from earlier assessments. However, a higher proportion of these referrals from recent assessments required medical investigation and/or treatment (11/14 compared to 18/31 of the referrals resulting from earlier assessments).

The frequency with which new abnormalities were documented by nursing staff was similar (25% and 29%). However, while new

Table 4.2. Comparison of the action taken as a result of new abnormal findings assessed using previous versions of the BPAF and the revised version of the BPAF

Category	Action taken in light of new abnormal findings (%)	
	Revised BPAF - June/July 1995	Previous versions of BPAF - Feb 1993 to Sept 1994
No documentation/ no action	59	41
Findings documented/ action taken	25	29
Referral made to other health professional	17	37
- unit doctor	14	31
- on-call SHO (urgent)	5	4
- referring medical team	0	7
- specialist medical review	1	1
- therapy staff	2	1

abnormalities assessed in earlier assessments using previous versions of the BPAF tended to be reported in the medical notes, those assessed using the revised BPAF tended to be documented in the nursing care plans.

Overall, the frequency with which new abnormalities assessed via the BPAF were acted on in some way by the nursing staff was higher in the earlier assessments using previous versions of the BPAF (59%) than in recent assessments using the revised BPAF (41%).

Summary

The evaluation of content validity focused on the adequacy of the techniques used to identify the total content domain and from this to select the most appropriate content for the BPAF.

The evaluation of the utilization of the BPAF has shown that a fair proportion of the BPAFs are completed each day. However, the frequency of completion of the recent assessments using the revised BPAF is lower than that of the earlier assessments using previous versions of the BPAF. A similar trend was found in the frequency of response to new abnormalities, with the influence of the BPAF on nurses' actions appearing to be higher for the earlier assessments with the previous versions of the BPAF than for the recent assessments using the revised BPAF.

Chapter 5
Discussion

This chapter discusses the implication of the findings of the reliability and validity testing of the BPAF.

Reliability of the BPAF

Here we discuss the meaning of the results of inter-rater reliability described in Chapter 3, addressing the nominal items first and then the ratio items. In examining these results it is not sufficient purely to consider the degree of agreement between assessors; there is also a need to examine the degree of disagreement and judge whether this would be clinically significant, i.e. would the difference in the assessment result in different actions by the nurse?

Nominal data

The percentage agreement and κ correlations of the assessments made by two independent assessors using the BPAF indicate that generally the inter-rater reliability of the BPAF is good. The total percentage agreement and κ correlation for all assessments in the study are 92% and 0.75 respectively, both of which fall easily within the acceptable levels of agreement specified by Waltz et al. (1991) and Altman (1991). The percentage agreement scores are all consistently higher than the κ correlations, as would be expected, as they do not account for the agreements made by chance. The inter-rater reliability of BPAF assessments conducted on the NLIU patients was found to be the highest in the study and not only remained stable over time but actually improved. This is demonstrated by comparing the scores achieved in period 1 (percentage agreement = 93% and κ = 0.76) and period 2 (percentage agreement = 94% and κ = 0.83) of assessments on the NLIU. The higher agreement in period 2 is likely to be due to assessors being more familiar with using the changed format of the BPAF.

The inter-rater reliability between novice and experienced assessors was the lowest in the study (percentage agreement = 89% and κ = 0.62), but still considered acceptable by Waltz et al. (1991) and good by Altman (1991). This shows that the use of the BPAF as an assessment tool can be easily and effectively taught and can help less experienced nurses to make similar assessments of patients as more experienced nurses. With the assumption that the experienced assessors are more accurate than the novice assessors, this also highlights the value of experience in the area of patient assessment.

The inter-rater reliability of two experienced assessors assessing patients on acute wards was also good (percentage agreement = 88% and κ = 0.72). Possible reasons why the reliability of these assessments was not as good as that of assessments conducted on the NLIU, also by two experienced assessors, are likely to be:

- less control over the time interval between assessments, because the timing of patient referral to the NLIU is often haphazard
- the numbers of assessments completed was much lower.

In examining the percentage agreement and κ scores of individual items on the BPAF, there are obvious variations in the degree of agreement between assessors. Items with consistently high scores included:

- bowels open
- catheterized
- purulent wound
- laboured/breathless
- slurred speech/dysarthric
- limb:weakness/flaccid.

Other items had consistently low scores and these included:

- pale skin
- rash
- dry mouth
- reduced tissue turgor
- cyanosis - peripheral
- visual disturbance.

Factors affecting the reliability of individual nominal items

There are several factors that appear to affect the reliability of items. One of the most important is the degree of subjective judgement involved in making the assessment. Only two items showed perfect agreement throughout the study and these are 'catheterized' and 'purulent wound'. These are items that are clear-cut to assess and therefore one would expect a high agreement. Other items involve a much greater degree of subjective judgement, for example assessing whether a patient is pale will involve making a judgement about what 'pale' looks like, which is difficult to quantify and therefore difficult to standardize.

Some patients were unclear and inconsistent in reporting their symptoms and often contradicted themselves. Possible reasons for this include:

- poor memory or understanding
- embarrassment about discussing certain symptoms, and urinary or bowel function, especially if the assessor was of the opposite sex (for the NLIU assessments one assessor was male and the other female)
- the significance they assign to the symptom, e.g. if a patient has had hip pain for over 20 years they may not report it because it is part of their 'normal life'.

For some items there was conflict between the patient's report and the assessor's observation, e.g. the patient said they had a dry mouth but on inspection it looked moist. In this situation disagreement between assessors is more likely. The method and extent of questioning used by the assessor may also affect the assessment made, e.g. a patient may say they do not feel dizzy when asked, but if this is explored further may admit to experiencing dizziness when first standing up.

The severity of the signs and symptoms are likely to affect the degree of agreement. When signs and symptoms are severe, agreement between assessors is much higher (Pinholt et al. 1987). When they are mild, they are often ambiguous and assessors are more likely to disagree. The patients who are suitable for the nurse-led service have been judged as 'medically stable' by the medical team who referred them to the NLIU and as such many of the signs and symptoms they experience are mild.

Ratio data

The standard deviation of the difference between assessors' scores, the tolerance interval of the difference between two assessors and the confidence interval for the mean of the difference between assessors' scores have all shown a surprisingly high level of inter-rater variability. The lower level of variability found between one novice and one expert assessor is possibly because they were more conscientious in the recording of the data. The novice assessors may have been more careful because the BPAF was new to them and the experienced assessor for these assessments was the author of this study, who therefore was likely to be particularly careful in collecting this data. The higher level of variability found between the two experienced assessors assessing patients on acute wards is likely to be due to the low number of assessments ($n = 8$) and the difficulty in controlling the time interval between the two assessments.

In examining these data for evidence of inter-rater reliability, the question of what degree of variability between assessors is acceptable must be considered. This requires some insight into what would constitute a clinically significant difference, i.e. would the difference in the assessment result in different actions by the nurse? Surprisingly, there was very little guidance on this in the literature. For temperature recording, Erickson (1980) and Fulbrook (1993) thought that differences in temperature recording of 0.2°C begin to have practical clinical importance, since in some situations they may affect the frequency of assessing temperature status and judgements about the need for treatment. Closs (1987) suggests that 'quite small changes in temperature could be highly clinically significant' for some patients, but fails to expand on what a 'quite small change' is and for which patients it would be clinically significant. Similarly, there is no indication of what a clinically significant difference would be for BP, heart rate and respiratory rate recording.

In examining the standard deviation of the difference between assessors' scores (s_{diff}) and the 95% tolerance intervals for the difference between the assessors' scores for the total number of assessments in the study, it can be seen that some of the differences would be clinically significant. The 95% tolerance interval for heart rate shows that for 95% of assessments made the scores of the two assessors would be within 20.81 beats/minute of each other. A difference of 20.81 beats/minute is almost certainly clinically significant in most people's resting heart rate. The 95% tolerance intervals for respiratory rate (8.01), diastolic BP (20.59), systolic BP (31.88) and temperature (0.85) also show that differences between assessors' recordings could be clinically significant.

Factors affecting the inter-rater reliability of ratio data

There are many documented factors that affect the reliability of recording of vital signs which are likely to have affected the assessments made in this study.

Blood pressure

Blood pressure naturally varies from moment to moment and has a circadian pattern, being lowest in early morning and highest in the early evening (Millar-Craig et al. 1978). Patients may find it stressful to have their blood pressure taken, which may lead to elevated results (Thompson 1981). If the patient's arm is not positioned at heart level and not supported, errors of up to 10 mmHg in both diastolic and systolic BP can occur (Mitchell et al. 1964). In some patients, particularly the elderly, there is a striking difference in the blood pressure when sitting, standing or lying down (Thompson 1981), and there can be differences of over 10 mmHg between arms (Kristensen 1982).

There are also various sources of error within the assessor, such as hearing acuity, effects of environmental noise (Walsh and Ford 1989) and the speed with which the assessor releases the pressure within the sphygmomanometer cuff (Thompson 1981). O'Brien and O'Malley (1979) found that assessors showed a strong preference for the terminal digits 0 and 5, even though a 5 mmHg mark does not appear on many scales. Conceicao et al. (1976) found that as many as half of the sphygmomanometers used in hospital are inaccurate.

Temperature

Temperature also has a diurnal pattern, being lowest in early morning and highest in early evening. The length of time taken to record an oral temperature is known to affect the recording obtained (Nichols and Verhonick 1968; Closs 1987). Failure to locate the thermometer in either of the sublingual pockets can lead to errors of up to −1.7°C in recorded temperature. Maintaining the thermometer in the correct position can be a problem for some patients, especially if they wear dentures (Beck and Campbell 1975). Hot and cold drinks can affect temperatures over a range from 1°C above to 3°C below actual temperature (Forster et al. 1970; Lee and Atkins 1972). Mouth breathing has been found to reduce temperature recordings (Erickson 1980).

Heart rate

Herbert (1989) identifies a lack of research in the area of heart rate recording. Heart rate varies from minute to minute and is affected by exercise, shock, excitement and anxiety. Although there was no support found in the literature, it could be questioned whether being assessed by a nurse of the opposite sex may affect heart rate recordings. It is interesting that a majority of the heart rate recordings in this study were even numbers, suggesting that the heart rate was probably not counted over a full minute as recommended in the 'definitions of items' table (see Appendix 9), which would introduce error in recordings.

Respiratory rate

Herbert (1989) also identifies a lack of research in the area of respiratory rate recording. As the patient can consciously control respiratory rate, the technique used to assess it is very important. Should the patient be aware that his or her breathing is being assessed, it may substantially affect the recording. Like the heart rate recordings, a majority of the respiratory rates recorded in this study were even numbers, suggesting that the respiratory rate may not have been assessed over a full minute.

All recordings of vital signs are also subject to assessor bias, with the assessor unconsciously biased towards raising or lowering according to his or her expectations of what the recordings should be. In addition, assessors may show a preference for certain conventional values, such as a blood pressure of 120/80 mmHg (Choi et al. 1978) or a respiratory rate of 20 breaths/minute (Walsh and Ford 1989).

The confidence intervals for the mean difference between assessors' scores (d) show that there was some bias between the assessors. This was demonstrated in respiratory rate and heart rate recordings. Bias between assessors was identified for temperature recordings conducted during period 2 of assessments on the NLIU and for diastolic BP recordings conducted by two experienced assessors on the acute wards. This bias suggests that there is some consistent difference between recordings obtained by two assessors, which is probably best explained by difference in recording technique used by the assessors.

Reliability of the BPAF as a whole

With the two different levels of measurement of data collected, i.e. nominal and ratio, it is not possible to get a measurement of reliability for the BPAF as a whole. By necessity the two types of data have to be assessed separately. The results discussed above indicate that there is generally good inter-rater reliability for the nominal data items of the BPAF. However, the inter-rater reliability of the ratio data items of the BPAF does not appear to be good, although guidance on what would be an acceptable agreement between assessors for data that is dynamic and can vary quickly from minute to minute was not available.

Validity of the BPAF

Content Validity

As discussed in Chapter 4, there are no objective methods to assess the adequacy of content coverage of an instrument, which, as a result, must be judged on the methods used to identify the ideal content for the instrument in line with its designated purpose. The methods used to revise the BPAF are those used and recommended by the studies reviewed in Chapter 1 and the well-known nursing research texts. The physical assessment literature was reviewed very thoroughly, which resulted in the tables of abnormal signs and symptoms for each physiological system (see Table 2.2 and Appendices 4 to 7). The experts were selected on the basis of their expertise and experience in physical assessment, assessment tool development and experience in using the BPAF. Changes were made to the BPAF and the definitions of its items in line with agreed suggestions from the group of experts. Therefore it is considered that content validity of the BPAF is supported. However, Chapter 2 gives a very detailed description of how the BPAF was revised, which should enable readers to make their own judgements.

Utilization of the BPAF

Frequency of completion

The frequency with which the BPAF is completed gives some insight into how effectively it fulfils its purpose. If it is rarely used then it will not be effective in helping the nursing staff to systematically assess patients. Findings have shown that 53% of earlier assessments and 32% of recent assessments using the revised BPAF were fully completed, and these figures rise to 71% and 52% respectively if partially completed assessments are included. Obviously 100% completion would be the ideal, but these figures do suggest that patients are likely to have a full systems-based assessment fairly frequently. It is interesting that the frequency of completion of the recent assessments using the revised BPAF is lower than that of the earlier assessments using previous versions of the BPAF. Possible reasons for the decrease in completion are:

- A large number of qualified staff vacancies on the unit during the data collection period, which places more pressure on staff and necessitates the use of temporary staff who are not familiar with the BPAF.

- Staff are no longer so anxious about the additional responsibility they carry and as a result of this are more comfortable with their role, relying less on the BPAF, which was viewed in the early stages of the nurse-led service as a 'safety net'.
- Patients appear to become acutely ill less frequently (shown by the reduction in referral back to the referring medical team, 7% in earlier assessments versus 0% in recent assessments) and as result, completion of the BPAF may be seen as less of a priority.

Action taken by nurses as a result of the detection of a new abnormality using the BPAF

Examination of the action taken by nursing staff as a result of the detection of a new abnormality using the BPAF gives a rudimentary view on how well the BPAF fulfils its purpose. If it rarely affects what nurses do as a result of identifying a new abnormality, then its effectiveness as an assessment tool must be in doubt. Findings have shown that the nurses acted in some way as a result of 59% of new abnormalities identified in earlier assessments and 41% of those identified in recent assessments using the revised BPAF. This illustrates that the instructions for use of the BPAF are not always followed, otherwise all new abnormal signs and symptoms would be at least documented in the medical or nursing notes. The frequency with which the BPAF influences nurses' actions appears to be higher for the earlier assessments with the previous versions of the BPAF than for the recent assessments using the revised BPAF. Possible reasons for this include:

- Documentation as a whole is less comprehensive because of staff shortages and the resulting time pressures on permanent staff.
- The new abnormal signs and symptoms identified were not considered significant enough to require action or documentation. Some of the items added to the first version of the BPAF and during this study reflect acute nursing needs, for example 'dry mouth', 'incontinence', 'reduced tissue turgour', 'joint/muscular pain' and 'reddening of pressure areas'. Changes in these signs and symptoms often varied from day to day and were frequently not documented other than on the BPAF. In the absence of documentation, action taken as a result of these assessments is unknown. However, this does suggest that these items are seen as less significant in terms of the purpose of the BPAF, which may be seen by nurses as predominantly 'medical'.
- Staff are less familiar with the BPAF, how to use it and its purpose.

The frequency of referrals made to medical staff as a result of the identification of new abnormal symptoms using the BPAF has also decreased in the recent assessments using the revised BPAF. Possible reasons for this include:

- Fewer of the abnormal signs and symptoms identified needed medical input.
- The nursing staff are better able to judge which abnormal signs and symptoms require medical input. This inference is supported by the higher proportion of unit doctor referrals from the recent assessments using the revised BPAF resulting in medical intervention.
- The type of patients transferred to the NLIU has changed over time and they are less likely to develop signs or symptoms that require medical input. This inference is supported by the absence of referrals back to the referring acute medical team as a result of recent assessments using the revised BPAF and the recent expansion of medically-led rehabilitation services available in the hospital, to which patients may be referred rather than to the NLIU.

The interpretation of these data has shown that both the completion of the BPAF and the degree of action by nurses in response to identification of abnormal symptoms is fair and as such demonstrates the potential of the tool in aiding assessment. Its full potential is difficult to judge until the reasons for non-compliance are explored further.

Strengths and limitations of the BPAF

Several strengths and limitations have been identified from both the findings of the study and the data collection process. Some of these strengths and limitations are inherent in the design of the assessment tool.

Strengths

One of the major strengths of the BPAF is that it is systematically structured and thus reduces the omission of assessment data collected. It is easy to use and does increase the documentation of patients' physical status. It does not take long to complete, about 10-15 minutes, and has been likened to an 'extended TPR chart'. Each of the items and how they are best assessed has been operationally defined (see Appendix 9) as recommended by Mallick (1981), although it cannot be assumed that these are used consistently. The assessment information is gained using more than one technique, direct observation and interviewing, which adds to its value (Mallick 1981).

Limitations

The BPAF, like any other assessment tool, is limited in its sphere of influence over the assessment made. It does not ensure that the assessment of each item is accurate, nor does it influence the nurses' interpersonal skills and perception, which are important in assessment (Hamers et al. 1994). Other than aiding the collection of the full range of information, it does not help the subsequent judgement made with the information collected. The dichotomous nature of the data collected is limiting. For instance, should a sign or symptom already present deteriorate, there is no way of indicating this deterioration on the BPAF. The amount of data collected using the BPAF may be misleading, as Elstein and Bordage (1988) suggest that collecting too much data may impair the nurse's ability to sort out and focus on the relevant variables. Some of the items on the BPAF rely on subjective judgement, and this can be seen as a limitation.

How findings relate to previous literature

The findings from this study do relate in some ways to previous literature concerning assessment, particularly in areas of clinical expertise, the process of assessment, documentation, the effect of models of care on care delivery and the question of how rigorous clinical assessment tools should be.

Clinical expertise

It was found that the level of agreement between experienced nurses using the BPAF tended to be higher than the level of agreement between an experienced and a novice assessor. Assuming that this increased agreement reflects an increased accuracy in the assessment made, then this coincides with the work of Benner (1984) and Corcoran (1986), who both concluded that experience is an important determinant of expertise. Tanner et al. (1987) found that with increased levels of knowledge and experience, there was a trend towards more systematic data collection and greater accuracy in diagnosis. In considering the findings of the action taken as a result of identifying abnormal signs and symptoms using the BPAF, some of the differences between the earlier assessments and the recent assessments could be due to the differences in the experience and knowledge of staff on the NLIU, as there had been many staff changes, particularly among senior staff, during the time between each set of assessments (i.e. September 1994 to May 1995).

Process of assessment

From some of the literature concerning assessment, particularly as part of the nursing process, the process of assessment would seem to be an uncomplicated task. However, in reality, it appears to be fraught with difficulty due to the high complexity and, at times, the ambiguity of assessment cues. The BPAF gives a simplistic view of assessment in that signs and symptoms are not always just present or absent. Although inter-rater agreement for dichotomous data is generally higher than for continuous data (Burns 1991), findings for the reliability testing of the nominal items of the BPAF have shown some degree of disagreement for some items that would appear uncomplicated to assess (e.g. 'irregular pulse', 'dizziness', 'special diet/feeding'), suggesting that no aspect of assessment can be assumed to be straightforward. Moreover Pinholt et al. (1987) found that clinicians were able to assess severe problems accurately but were poor at recognizing moderate problems. Elstein and Bordage (1988) suggest that excessive data collection may impair the clinician's ability to sort out and focus on relevant variables, which suggests that the BPAF as a routine assessment tool may complicate decision making.

Documentation

The degree of completion of the BPAF and the action taken as a result of identifying a new abnormal symptom show that while the BPAF was designed to improve documentation of patient assessment, it has not been used to its greatest potential and highlights the difficulty in designing documentation to be used by nurses. The issue of the burden of paperwork has been a perennial problem in nursing for a long time (de la Cuesta 1983; NPEWG 1986).

The effect of a model of care on care delivery.

With the apparent decrease in utilization of the BPAF over the time it has been in use, it can be questioned whether its conceptual basis is still congruous with the values of the nursing team. Pearson and Vaughan (1986) imply that team agreement on the most appropriate way to give care in a particular area will increase continuity of care patterns. Reed and Bond (1991) found that nursing care was confined within an inappropriate model, and similarly it is possible that the BPAF is perceived to be a predominantly 'medical' tool to be used for identification of potential medical problems. Initially this was its most prominent aim. However, as a result of the first revision using Majesky et al.'s work the BPAF was intended to reflect acute nursing as well as acute medical needs, an aim that staff may not be aware of. With the reduction of medical referrals made and changes in the type of patient referred, it is possible that the BPAF is seen as less of a priority. It would appear that the BPAF has not been well integrated into the rest of the documentation system and the information gained from its use does not seem to influence nursing care plans. For example, should a patient be assessed as having a dry mouth or reduced tissue turgor, this generally did not result in a documented nursing plan to increase fluid intake. Possibly the use of two models of care, i.e. Roper et al. and the 'medical' model has caused tension within the overall service.

How rigorous should clinical assessment tools be?

In conducting this study, a difficulty has been identified in the level of rigour expected and desired in clinical assessment tools. For research tools, reliability and validity are essential and observers are highly trained to minimize observer bias in data collection. However, in clinical practice, the same strict procedures are not upheld and are more difficult to achieve. Generally, clinical assessment tools are seen as guides only and not procedures to be followed with any consistency (Mayers 1978; Marriner 1979). There are differing opinions about how rigorous clinical practice should be. Mallick (1981) thinks that rigour in clinical tools is as important as in research tools, in order to facilitate rational care planning and further nursing at a theoretical level. Contrary to this, Kitson (1987) argues that nurses must start to rely less on the scientific and objective protocols that have confined nursing and focus more on the individual patient and the more personal aspects of nursing. While this study does not attempt to add to this philosophical debate, it does highlight the variability in nurses' assessments, especially in vital signs for which there is no 'benchmark' to judge how acceptable the variability is.

Limitations of the study

The study had several limitations. The limited time and resources available meant that the number of patients studied was lower than would have been ideal to test the reliability and utilization of the BPAF. The low occurrence of some of the signs and symptoms has limited assessment of inter-rater reliability. There was difficulty in timing the assessments on acute wards because of the service requirements, and at times this caused the time intervals between assessments to be longer than planned. The extent to which this influenced the findings cannot be known. While not thought to be necessary at the time, reliability of the BPAF may have been improved by having a discussion session for the experienced assessors to standardize methods of assessment, especially for vital signs which have shown surprising variability. A large limiting factor to testing the BPAF was the depleted staffing levels on the ward, which compromises all activities and must be taken into account when considering the utilisation of the BPAF findings. It was not the best time to test the BPAF to see its full potential.

Conclusion

To conclude, all four aims of the study have been addressed. The BPAF has been scrutinized and revised in a way that supports its content validity. Inter-rater reliability of the nominal items of the BPAF was found to be good and although the inter-rater reliability of the ratio items appear disappointing, no guidance on how to judge the clinical significance of the variability was found. With relatively little teaching, novice assessors were able to use the BPAF and achieve good inter-rater reliability with experienced assessors, although this was lower than inter-rater reliability between two experienced assessors, indicating that experience does affect assessment skills. In examining patient assessment documentation retrospectively, rate of completion and evidence of action taken in response to assessment of a new abnormal sign or symptom was found to be fair, showing that the BPAF does affect the actions of the nurses, although it could be utilized more. However, in examining these data, the depleted staffing level particularly at senior level must be considered.

These findings have several implications for the NLIU. When new staff are recruited it would seem to be of utmost importance to review the 'model' of nursing held by the team and the place the BPAF has within this. The method of assessment of items with lower inter-rater reliability needs to be closely examined to reduce this variability. The BPAF has been shown to add structure to assessment and influence nurses' actions to some extent and, as such, has implications for nursing assessment outside the NLIU. It is a useful teaching tool for physical assessment. With the reduction in junior doctors' hours, it may become more useful by increasing the comprehensiveness of nurses' assessment and thus allowing the early identification of patient deterioration. Similarly it may be useful in the community as part of an early discharge initiative. However, it is important to acknowledge that in addition to the potential benefit of systematic assessment facilitated by the BPAF, there is also a danger that the BPAF will become another of the 'rituals' described by Walsh and Ford (1989), such as 'doing the obs'. Nurses may start to think of it as an end in itself and stop thinking about the information it produces.

Suggestions for further research

If use of the BPAF is to be extended to other areas, its reliability and utilization testing would need to be replicated with larger numbers. Further research to examine the feasibility of a meaningful scoring system would add to its scope and may enable more comprehensive validity testing. The exploration of individual item severity scoring would add to its usefulness. To test its effectiveness as a tool to promote systematic assessment and allow early identification of patient deterioration, it would be interesting to conduct a randomized controlled trial in the community with chronically ill patients who require frequent hospital admission to assess whether regular use of the BPAF by a community nurse would reduce frequency of admission. A similar study could be conducted with patients participating in an early discharge initiative, to investigate whether the use of the BPAF would be beneficial in prevention of readmission.

To consider the finding that the BPAF can be easily taught to nurses with no experience of using it to the extent that their inter-rater reliability with experienced nurses is good, it would be interesting to explore and evaluate its use as a physical assessment teaching tool.

It can therefore be seen that the BPAF could prove to be a valuable tool worth developing for use in several areas of nursing: teaching, clinical practice and, should a scoring system be devised, possibly patient outcome research.

Appendix 1
Physical assessment teaching information for staff

Guidelines for physical assessment

The aims of the daily physical assessment are:

1. to detect abnormalities and changes in the patient's condition early so that appropriate action can be taken
2. to have a systematic picture of the patient to assist in presenting problems in a structured manner if medical intervention is required
3. to document findings in a concise manner.

The first assessment is done when the patient arrives on the ward. This initial assessment is very important. It provides a baseline against which later changes can be measured. This first assessment is the responsibility of the nurse who admits the patient. If the nurse admitting the patient does not feel confident in doing this examination, it is his or her responsibility to ask an experienced member of staff to do this assessment as soon as possible.

How to carry out a physical examination

This may seem a daunting task at first but only by doing it will competence and confidence develop.

Start the examination by looking at the patient. Assess general appearance. Look for changes. Look at colour. Is the patient pale, flushed, cyanosed, dehydrated? Does the patient look in pain?

One of the best ways to carry out a physical examination is to develop a systematic approach. What this means is that each system is reviewed individually. This will enable you to carry in your mind the pattern the examination will follow.

Review of systems. (The assessment forms on the ward are structured to enable this method to be followed.)

Cardiovascular system

- Make sure patient is at 45°
- Look for signs of:
  – cyanosis
  – dyspnoea
- Assess ankle oedema. This is done by gently pressing over the tibia for a few seconds to see if pitting of the skin occurs
- Assess radial pulse note regularity/irregularity. If there is irregularity do apex beat as well
- Assess blood pressure
- Enquire about:
  – dizzy spells
  – chest pain
  – palpitations
- Abnormal findings:
  – chest pains – ask patient to describe it. Is it related to exertion? Is it relieved by position/eating?
  – irregular heart rate – request or do urgent ECG
  – ankle oedema – suggests heart failure. Do daily weights. Monitor fluid intake and output

Respiratory system

- First look at breathing pattern. Look for signs of distressed breathing, e.g. the use of accessory muscles. Count respiratory rate
- If there is dypnoea enquire into:
  – when it began
  – is it worse on exertion?
  – is it relieved by position, e.g. sitting up/lying down?
- Cough – is it dry or productive?
- Sputum – assess colour, quantity. Greenish sputum suggests infection. White frothy sputum suggests heart failure
- Assess breath sounds. Always listen even if you are unsure of findings. The more you listen the more you learn and become confident. Ask for a second opinion
  – normal breath sounds/vesicular
  – inspiration/expiration
  – expiration is shorter than inspiration and there is no gap between the two phases
  – added sounds. There are three added sounds:
    1. wheeze as in asthma and chronic bronchitis
    2. crackles/crepitations (rales). These are bubbling noises.

Crackles are coarser than crepitations and are typically heard in cases of infection. Crepitations are very fine and are a sign of pulmonary oedema

3. pleural rub. This is a creaking sound heard when the inflamed pleura rub together

- Abnormal findings:
  - greenish sputum – send specimen. Sign of infection
  - coarse crackles – suggest chest infection. Monitor temperature
  - fine crepitations – suggest heart failure. Look for other signs, e.g. ankle oedema, dyspnoea. Monitor weight, intake/output. Ask for second opinion

Gastrointestinal

- Assess appetite. Look at food chart
- Look at mouth and tongue (dry, coated). Dry tongue suggests dehydration. Monitor fluid intake
- Enquire about:
  - nausea
  - bowel pattern – diarrhoea/constipation
  - shape, look, distension
- Inspect abdomen – inquire about abdominal pain. Look for tenderness. Ask patient to describe where the pain is and the duration. Is it relieved by anything, e.g. eating, change of position. What does it feel like, e.g. dull, colicky. Palpation – if you have to palpate be very gentle. Look for masses
- Types of abdominal pains:
  - waxing and waning pains = intestinal obstruction
  - acute colicky = enteric infection
  - chronic = peptic ulcer disease
  - dull = constipation

Genitourinary

- Assess urinary changes:
  - dysuria
  - frequency
  - output
  - colour
  - odour
  - incontinence
- Look for loin pains.
- Abnormal findings:
  - dysuria frequency – send MSU, monitor temperature, monitor fluid intake/output
  - concentrated urine – monitor intake/output

Central nervous system

- Assess alertness, conscious level, drowsiness, agitation, confusion
- Assess behaviour – appropriate or inappropriate
- Look for signs of:
  - headache
  - blurred/double vision
  - abnormal sensation, e.g. numbness, tingling
- Assess speech – coherence, slurring
- Assess muscle power – weakness

General points to remember

- Always document abnormal findings and the plan of action. Follow through the documentation so that it is clear how and when the problem has been resolved
- Note tests and dates
- To assist your decision making look for other symptoms. For example, if there is ankle oedema, assess chest for fine crepitations, or if patient is pyrexial look for other symptoms, such as pain, cough, frequency of urine
- For patients on digoxin, warfarin, phenytoin, aminophylline, monitor levels. Be guided by the unit doctor/pharmacist as to when to do levels.
- Monitor FBC in patients at risk of GI bleed or known to have had GI bleed, or with a history of low haemoglobin
- Monitor urea and electrolytes in patients with poor hydration, hypertension, UTI, long-term infection, diarrhoea, heart failure
- In patients with history of congestive heart failure, monitor daily weights
- In patients who show signs of confusion:
  - send MSU
  - monitor intake/output
  - monitor temperature
- Do ECG if patient complains of chest pains or has an irregular heart rate

(Sadie Collison 1994)

Appendix 2
Second version of the NLIU Physical Assessment Framework

DAILY PATIENT ASSESSMENT

Nursing Development Unit

Patient Name..
Hospital Number...................................
Primary Nurse...

Week beginning...........................

		M	T	W	T	F	S	S
O	Respiration: rate (normal 12–18)*							
X	laboured							
Y	other abnormality							
G	Cough							
E	Sputum							
N	Moist							
A	Wheeze							
T	Pulse: rate*							
I	irregular							
O	weak							
N	Chest pain							
	Pitting oedema							
	Calf pain							
	Dizziness on standing							
F								
O	Reduced tissue turgour							
O	Dry mouth							
D	Coated mouth							
+								
F	Weekly weight*							
L	Nausea							
U	Poor appetite							
I	Dysphagia							
D	Special diet/feeding*							
	Concentrated urine							
	Odour							

E	Pain on micturition							
L	Frequency							
I	Incontinent							
M	Catheterized*							
	Bowels open*							
	Constipated stool							
	Loose stool							
	Faecal incontinence							
	Body temperature							
	Skin: hot							
	cool							
S	Cyanotic – central							
K	Cyanotic – peripheral							
I	Pale							
N	Jaundice							
	Reddening of pressure areas							
	Ulceration/damage							
	Purulent wound							
	Limb: weakness/flaccid							
	contracture/spasticity							
N	Tingling							
E	Visual disturbance							
U	Lethargic							
R	Disorientated							
O	Slurred/dysarthric							
	Dysphasic							

This document is to assist you in providing a daily picture of your patient. Please complete starred items and sign against other relevant items. Any new abnormal finding will need action/referral documented. June 1994

Appendix 3
First version of the NLIU Physical Assessment Framework.

Patient Name............................ Hospital Number.....................
Primary Nurse...........................
Week beginning...............................

		M	T	W	T	F	S	S
TIME:								
	Unlaboured							
	Laboured							
	Other abnormality							
R	Rate: normal (12–18)							
E	rapid							
S	Sounds: clear							
P	moist							
	cough							
	stridor							
	wheeze							
	Pulse: regular							
C	irregular							
I	strong							
R	weak							
C	Chest pain							
	Pitting oedema							
	Normal voiding							
	Incontinent							
	Pain on micturition							
E	Frequency							
L	Odour							
I	Bowels open							
M	Bowels not open							
	Faecal incontinence							
	Loose stool							
	Constipated stool							

	Temperature: warm										
	hot										
S	cool										
K	Colour: pink										
I	cyanotic										
N	pale										
	jaundice										
	Oedema										
	Alert										
N	Lethargic										
E	Orientated										
U	Disorientated										
R	Normal power										
O	Weakness										
	Tingling										
	Visual disturbance										
S											
P	Clear										
E	Slurred										
E	Inappropriate										
C	Dysphasic										
H											

Guide for completion

This form should be placed in the medical notes and used every day after the gathering of baseline data. The most senior nurse caring for the patient should assess the patient and initial against the relevant categories. If a category in a bold box is appropriate, further documentation of assessment and action should be placed in the medical notes and any appropriate referrals made. Any further change should be documented and action taken accordingly.

Jan 1993

Appendix 4
Abnormal physiological signs and symptoms of the cardiovascular system

	Munro and Edwards (1990)	Toghill (1995)	Bates (1995)	Turner and Blackwood (1991)	Hayes and MacWalter (1992)
Principal symptom	4 specified (first 4 items)	5 specified (first 5 items)	none specified	none specified	none specified
Symptoms and signs of abnormal function (those in bold are items on the BPAF before this study. Those in italics are those added during the study)	- **dyspnoea** - **chest pain** - **oedema** - *palpitations* - **cough** - **frothy sputum** - **pallor** - **skin temperature** - *clammy skin* - altered state of consciousness - syncope - **excessive tiredness** - **nausea and vomiting** - **diarrhoea** (digoxin toxicity) - reduced urine output - signs of DVT: **pain,** *swelling,* pale or very red, warm - **cyanosis, peripheral or central** - **abnormal pulse rate**	- **chest pain** - **breathlessness** - **ankle swelling** - *palpitations* - **dizziness/blackouts** - **pallor** - **skin temperature** - *clammy skin* - **nausea** - reduced consciousness - **white/pink frothy sputum** - **cough** - **wheeze** - **cyanosis peripheral/central** - **pyrexia** - **irregular pulse/heart rhythm** - **abnormal pulse rate, e.g. tachycardia, bradycardia** - **pulse volume** - *abnormal BP* - raised JVP	- **abnormal heart rate** - **irregular heart rhythm** - *abnormal blood pressure* - **chest pain** - *palpitations* - **dyspnoea** - **oedema** - abnormal carotid pulse - raised JVP - abnormal apex beat and position - abnormal heart sounds - additional heart sounds and murmurs	- **chest pain** - **breathlessness** - **ankle swelling** - **palpitations** - **cough** - **frothy sputum** - **blood in sputum** - blackouts - **cyanosis, central/peripheral** - **abnormal pulse rate** - **irregular pulse/heart rhythm** - **abnormal pulse volume** - abnormal pulse waveform - *abnormal BP* - raised JVP - abnormal position of apex pulse - abnormal heart sounds - additional heart sounds and murmurs	- **pallor** - sweating - **cyanosis** - **breathlessness** - **peripheral oedema** - signs of DVT: *swelling* associated with redness, **tenderness,** including skin temperature - abnormal position of apex beat - **skin temperature** - **abnormal pulse rate** - **irregular pulse** - abnormal pulse character - **abnormal pulse volume** - *abnormal BP* - raised JVP - hepatomegaly - abnormal heart sounds

	- **irregular pulse rate** - abnormal pulse character and **volume** - *abnormal BP* - raised JVP - abnormal position of apex beat	- signs of DVT: *leg swelling*, **calf pain** (+ Homan's sign), warmth, discolouration - **basal crackles on lung auscultation** - cardiomegaly - hepatomegaly - position of cardiac apex - abnormal heart sounds - additional heart sounds, e.g. murmurs, clicks, snaps		- **basal crepitations on lung auscultation** - enlarged tender liver - **pyrexia** - weak or absent peripheral pulses	- additional heart sounds and murmurs - **crepitations on lung auscultation**
Normal values Heart rate	50-100/min	40/min(athletes)-200/min (young people with marked emotional or physical stress)	60-100/min	50-100/min	60-100/min - physiological variation
Blood pressure	not specified	not specified	- normal <130/<85 - high normal 130-139/85-89 - mild hypertension 140-149/90-99 - moderate hypertension 150-159/100-109 - severe hypertension 160-179/110-119 - very severe hypertension >210/>120	- 165/95 is considered to be hypertension - a wide pulse pressure, e.g. 160/30 suggests aortic incompetence - a narrow pulse pressure, e.g. 95/80 suggests aortic stenosis - a difference of >20 mm systolic between arms suggests arterial occlusion, e.g. dissecting aneurysm	not specified

Appendix 5
Abnormal physiological signs and symptoms of the neurological system

	Munro and Edwards (1990)	Toghill (1995)	Bates (1995)	Turner and Blackwood (1991)	Hayes and MacWalter (1992)
Principal symptoms	None specified	6 common presenting symptoms identified (first 6 items)	None specified	None specified	None specified. This system not dealt with as a whole but rather as particular dysfunctions
Symptoms and signs of abnormal function (those in bold are items on the BPAF before this study. Those in italics are those added during the study)	General - *headaches* - **visual disturbance** - *fits* - *faints - vertigo* - **tingling** - *numbness (paraesthesiae)* - **muscle weakness** - hearing symptoms, e.g. deafness, tinnitus - excessive thirst - neck stiffness - **pyrexia** - sleep patterns - *mood changes* - ***micturition disturbance*** - intellectual deterioration - **disorientation** - **dysphasia** - **dysarthria** - dysphonia	General - blackouts - *headaches* - **visual disturbance** - *dizziness* - **paralysis/weakness** and difficulty walking - **confusion** - **nausea** - neck stiffness - **pyrexia** - abnormal gait/posture - **dysphasia**, expressive and receptive - **disorientated** - memory impairment - personality changes - **dysarthria** - **dysphagia** - dyspraxia/apraxia	General - *headaches* - fainting - blackouts - seizures - **weakness** - **paralysis** - *numbness* - **tingling** - tremors - involuntary movements - **lethargy** - coma - **abnormal breathing pattern** - **abnormal pulse**, *BP*, **temperature** Cranial nerves - **abnormal visual acuity/visual fields** - abnormal pupil reactions	General - *abnormal behaviour, e.g. restless, agitated* - *abnormal emotional state, e.g. euphoric, hostile* - **impaired conscious level** - *confusion* - **disorientation, e.g. to time, place, person** - **abnormal speech: slurred, dysarthria,** dysphonia, **dysphasia/aphasia** - apraxia - agnosia - memory impairment - *headache* - **blurred or double vision** - **dizziness**	Stroke - **hemiparesis or hemiplegia** - **impaired consciousness** - abnormal gait - abnormal posture - **abnormal motor function, i.e. reduced power, altered tone,** impaired co-ordination, and altered reflexes - abnormal sensory function, i.e. sensory loss (light touch, pin-prick and temperature), altered proprioception - apraxia - **dysarthria** - **dysphasia/aphasia**

Cranial nerves - abnormal sense of smell - abnormal visual acuity/visual fields - abnormal ocular movements - abnormal pupillary reflexes - facial muscle weakness/loss of sensation - abnormal corneal reflex - impaired facial movement - deafness - impaired gag reflex - impaired palatial movement and reflex - abnormal movement of the tongue Motor system - dypraxia/apraxia - **paralysis/weakness** - co-ordination impairment - **changes in muscle tone, e.g. hypotonia, hypertonia, spasticity, rigidity**	Motor system - signs of muscle wasting - **changes in muscle tone, e.g. hypotonia, hypertonia, spasticity, rigidity** - **reduced muscle power** - impaired co-ordination - abnormal involuntary movements - abnormal tendon reflexes, e.g. biceps, triceps, knee, ankle, and plantar **Sensory system** - *pain* - *numbness* - *altered sensation or paraesthesiae* - impaired sensation of: light touch, vibration, position, pain, temperature - abnormal two point discrimination Cranial nerves - anosmia (associated with loss of taste) - **abnormal visual acuity/visual fields, e.g. double vision**	- abnormal extra-ocular movements - abnormal corneal reflexes - facial muscle weakness - impaired hearing - **swallowing difficulty** - palatal paralysis - impaired gag reflex - **dysarthria** Motor system - **hemiplegic posture** - involuntary muscle movements - signs of muscle atrophy - **altered muscle tone, e.g. spasticity, rigidity and flaccidity** - **muscle weakness** - impaired co-ordination - abnormal gait - poor proprioception Sensory system - impaired touch, temperature, pain and vibration sensation	- unsteady or abnormal gait - **weakness** - *numbness* - **'pins and needles' sphincter disturbance** - *depression* - *anxiety* - sleep disturbance - fits or faints Cranial nerves - impaired ability to smell - **impaired visual acuity/visual fields** - abnormal pupil reactions/size - abnormal external ocular movements, ptosis, nystagmus - impaired corneal reflex - jaw muscle weakness - facial muscle weakness - impaired gag reflex - **impaired swallowing** - palatal weakness	- **dysphagia** - agnosia Confused patient - *delirium* - **disorientation to time, place, and person** - impaired short-term memory - *altered mood* - emotional lability - *hypotension* - presence of primitive reflexes - **drowsiness** - **pyrexia - presence of infection** - **crackles - presence of infection** Eyes - proptosis - ptosis - abnormal pupils, i.e. size, shape, symmetry and reactivity - **visual field abnormality** - abnormal eye movements, e.g. nystagmus

Munro and Edwards (1990)	Toghill (1995)	Bates (1995)	Turner and Blackwood (1991)	Hayes and MacWalter (1992)
- abnormal involuntary movements/tremor - hypokinesis - abnormal posture/gait - muscle wasting Sensory system - pain (commonly burning or stabbing) - numbness - altered sensation or paraesthesiae, e.g. 'pins and needles' - impaired sensation of: light touch, pain, temperature, position vibration - abnormal two-point discrimination - abnormal reflexes, e.g. biceps, triceps, supinator, abdominals, knee, ankle, plantar	- abnormal pupillary responses/size - abnormal eye movement - absent corneal reflex - jaw muscle weakness - abnormal facial muscle weakness/contraction - nerve deafness - **dysphagia** - dysphonia - **dysarthria** - impaired gag reflex - palatal weakness	- impaired stereognosis, number identification and two-point discrimination - abnormal reflexes, e.g. biceps, triceps, supinator, abdominals, knee, ankle, plantar	Motor system - abnormal gait/posture - involuntary muscle movements - signs of muscle wasting - impaired co-ordination - **altered muscle tone** - **reduced muscle power** - impaired tendon reflexes - retention of urine Sensory system - impaired sensation of: vibration, position, pain, light touch, temperature, two-point discrimination	Cranial nerves (excluding II, III, IV & VI - eyes) - anosmia - jaw muscle weakness - abnormal corneal reflex - abnormal facial sensation - abnormal facial muscle contraction/weakness - abnormal hearing - abnormal gag and palatal reflex - asymmetrical palatal movement - **dysphagia** - dysphonia

Appendix 6
Abnormal physiological signs and symptoms of the gastrointestinal system

	Munro and Edwards (1990)	Toghill (1995)	Bates (1995)	Turner and Blackwood (1991)	Hayes and MacWalter (1992)
Principal symptoms	10 specified (first 10 items)	Not specified	Not specified	Not specified	Not specified
Symptoms and signs of abnormal function (those in bold are items on the BPAF before this study. Those in italics are those added during the study)	- **impaired appetite** - **difficulty in swallowing** - **heartburn** - *abdominal pain* - **nausea** - *vomiting* - *weight loss* - *gastrointestinal bleeding* - **alteration in bowel habit** - **jaundice** - *rigidity of abdominal muscles, localized and generalized* - *enlarged, tender liver on palpation* - *enlarged spleen* - *abnormal sounds on auscultation, e.g. gas sounds resonant, shifting dullness with ascites* - *increased frequency of bowel sounds, e.g.*	- *pain* - **nausea** - *vomiting* - **difficulty in swallowing** - **change in bowel habit** - *blood and/or mucus in motion* - **diarrhoea** - *steatorrhoea* - *melaena* - **heartburn** - *excessive wind* - *absence of bowel sounds* - *enlarged, tender liver on palpation* - *abnormal liver shape* - *enlarged spleen* - **jaundice** - *spider naevi* - *abnormal sounds on auscultation, e.g. gas sounds resonant, shifting dullness with ascites*	- **trouble swallowing** - **heartburn** - **reduced appetite** - **nausea** - *vomiting* - *regurgitation* - *haematemesis* - *indigestion* - **change in bowel habit** - *abnormal colour of motions* - **frequency of bowel movements** - *passing blood/melaena* - *haemorrhoids* - **constipation** - **diarrhoea** - *abdominal pain* - *excessive wind* - **jaundice** - *increased/decreased bowel sounds*	- **nausea** - *vomiting* - **trouble swallowing** - *indigestion* - *abdominal pain* - **alteration in bowel habit** - **diarrhoea** - *blood/mucus in stool* - *steatorrhoea* - *melaena* - **hypotension/drowsiness** in GI bleed - **jaundice** - *spider naevi* - **dry tongue** - **diminished skin turgor** - *abdominal distension* - *symmetrical or asymmetrical* - *guarding (a reflex action to protect from pain)* - **pyrexia**, e.g. in peritonitus	- **jaundice** - **dry tongue** - *oral candida* - *spider naevi* - *abdominal distension* - *symmetrical or asymmetrical* - *pain and tenderness* - *increased abdominal muscle tone and guarding* - *presence of abnormal masses* - *enlarged, tender liver* - *enlarged spleen* - *shifting dullness/hyper-resonance on percussion* - *altered bowel sounds particularly loud high-pitched and 'tinkling'* - *altered frequency of bowel sounds, e.g. absent, diminished or increased*

	in enteritis, presence of blood in bowel or mechanical obstruction - high pitched tinkling bowel sounds in obstruction - absent bowel sounds, e.g. paralytic ileus		- abnormal proportions and patterns of tympany and dullness on percussion - abdominal guarding with tenderness - presence of abnormal masses - enlarged, tender liver - enlarged spleen	- enlarged, tender liver - **drowsiness** in hepatic encephalopathy - enlarged spleen - presence of abnormal masses - shifting dullness/hyper-resonance on percussion - absence of bowel sounds - hyperactive bowel sounds or 'tinkling'	
Normal values - frequency of bowel sounds	- gurgling heard every 5-10 seconds	- not specified	- not specified	- not specified	varies considerably but >30/min is usually abnormal
- frequency of bowel movement	- not specified	- varies in the individual from 2-3/day to 2-3/week	- not specified	- not specified	- not specified

Appendix 7
Abnormal physiological signs and symptoms of the genitourinary system

	Munro and Edwards (1990)	Toghill (1995)	Bates (1995)	Turner and Blackwood (1991)	Hayes and MacWalter (1992)
Principal symptoms	Not specified	Not specified	Not specified	Not specified	Not specified
Symptoms and signs of abnormal function (those in bold are items on the BPAF before this study. Those in italics are those added during the study) There is a difference in these texts as to what constitutes the genitourinary system. Toghill describes sexually transmitted diseases only, whereas Turner and Blackwood describe urinary and menstrual symptoms as well	- loin pain - **burning pain on micturition (dysuria)** - **increased frequency of micturition** - haematuria In men: - *reduction in force of stream* - *hesitancy* - *terminal dribbling* - scrotal swelling In women: - **stress incontinence** - vaginal discharge - disturbance in menstrual period	The kidneys and bladder - loin pain - ureteric colic - poluria - nocturia - **frequency with small volumes** - *difficulty in micturition* - **pain on micturition** - oliguria (<400 ml/day) - anuria - retention of urine - haematuria - **incontinence** - **urgency** - cloudy urine - **odorous urine** - proteinuria - glucosuria/ketouria - **weight loss** - **dehydration** - **rapid respiration (Kussmaul's breathing)**	Urinary - **frequency of urination** - polyuria - nocturia - **burning or pain on urination** - haematuria - urgency - reduction of force of stream - hesitancy - **incontinence** In men: - urethral discharge - testicular pain or masses In women: - vaginal discharge - vulval itching - disturbance in menstrual period - heavy menstrual bleeding - bleeding between periods and after menopause	- loin pain - *nocturia* - *difficulty passing urine* - haematuria - polyuria In men: - *slow onset of micturition* - *poor stream* - *terminal dribbling* In women: - disturbance in menstrual period - heavy menstrual bleeding - bleeding between periods or after menopause - vaginal discharge	Uraemia - **drowsiness** - **deep sighing breaths** - **rapid, shallow breaths** - hiccoughs - muscle tremor - pruritus - excessive bruising - **periorbital oedema at night** - **ankle oedema during the day** - raised JVP - **diminished skin turgor** (where there is a pre-renal component) - enlarged kidneys on palpation - pericardial rub on auscultation

- generalized twitching of muscles - **drowsiness** -itchiness of skin <u>Genitourinary medicine</u> - genital skin rashes In men: - urethral discharge - dysuria In women: - vaginal discharge - vulval irritation	- enlarged kidneys on palpation - costovertebral tenderness	- **basal crepitations on lung auscultation** - cloudy urine - **dark urine (concentrated or contains blood)** - proteinuria - glucosuria

Appendix 8
Definition of items on the Byron Physical Assessment Framework before refinement by expert group

Item on physical assessment framework	Definition
Respiration: rate (normal 12–18)	Number of full breaths, i.e. inspiration and expiration phases counted in one full minute. Should be done in such a way that the patient is not aware of what you are doing
laboured	'An uncomfortable awareness of the need to breathe' (Toghill 1995). Use of accessory muscles of respiration by which the whole thoracic cage is, in effect, lifted off the diaphragm with every breath. Patient may have difficulty talking due to breathlessness
other abnormality	e.g. stridor
Cough	A cough involves making a forced expiratory effort against a closed glottis, which suddenly opens resulting in an explosive release of air carrying with it respiratory secretions. The cough reflex is stimulated by material in the airway lumen and events in the airway wall
Sputum	Patients may not know the term 'sputum', 'phlegm' may be better. Sputum is a respiratory tract secretion produced with certain conditions. Can be serous (clear, watery or frothy, e.g. in pulmonary oedema), mucoid (clear, grey or white, e.g. in chronic bronchitus/chronic asthma) or purulent (yellow, green or brown, e.g. in pulmonary infection)
Moist	Refers to the presence of crackles (intermittent, non-musical, short sounds) in lung fields on auscultation. Fine crackles are soft, high in pitch and very brief (sounds like rice crispies). Coarse crackles are somewhat louder, lower in pitch and not quite so brief. Late inspiratory crackles are usually fine and heard in dependent portions of the lungs, and causes include pulmonary oedema
Wheeze	Described as musical sounds produced by the passage of air through narrowed airways. Invariably louder during expiration and often confined to that part of the respiratory cycle. Is a cardinal symptom of airflow obstruction
Pulse: rate	Generally the radial pulse is taken as a measurement of heart rate, although in some situations they may not be the same. Pulse rate value is generally assumed to denote number of heartbeats per minute. Pulse should be assessed over a minute to ensure that any irregularities and abnormalities have been assessed
irregular	Can be regularly or irregularly irregular. The normal pulse should be of regular, even rhythm and volume. Should the pulse be irregular in any way the apex beat should also be assessed for rate and rhythm and any

	deficit between the apex and radial beats determined
weak	Generally the pulse is said to be weak when it is difficult to palpate, i.e. the rise and fall of the blood vessel feels faint under the finger. Systolic BP of 50 mmHg required to palpate a femoral or brachial pulse and needs to be higher to palpate a radial pulse
Chest pain	Assessed by patient report. Can be due to cardiac ischaemia, where patients often describe chest pain that is 'tight', 'pressing', or 'crushing'. It frequently radiates to the left arm and less frequently to the right arm, back, neck, jaw and teeth. Important non-cardiac chest pain includes pleuritic pain (sharp, stabbing pain aggravated by breathing/coughing), musculoskeletal pain (continuous and dull ache) and heartburn (substernal burning pain often confused with cardiac pain)
Pitting oedema	Occurs when fluid collects in the loose tissues of the feet and ankles (or sacrum if patient is lying in bed). Oedema occurs when the venous pressure plus the hydrostatic pressure of the upright posture exceeds the oncotic pressure of the plasma. In the presence of pitting oedema, an imprint of the fingers will be left when the area is pressed firmly, as the fluid in the tissues is displaced and will gradually fill in when the pressure is released. Common causes are heart failure and low plasma albumen, in which case the ankle swelling is symmetrical. In cases when ankle swelling is asymmetrical it is likely to be due to DVT or reduced muscle tone in the weak leg as a result of a CVA
Calf pain	Assessed by patient report. Unilateral calf pain is often caused by DVT. Pain occurs when the muscle mass containing the affected vein is squeezed. In the presence of a venous thrombosis of the calf, sharp dorsiflexion of the foot will be painful (Homan's sign). Other associated signs of DVT are unilateral swelling of the leg, warmth and discoloration, although all these signs are not very reliable
Dizziness on standing	Assessed by patient report. Patients often describe dizziness as giddiness, floating on air, faintness or light-headedness. Common causes include anaemia, postural hypotension, dehydration or phenytoin toxicity
Reduced tissue turgor	Loss of elasticity of the skin can be a sign of dehydration and can be demonstrated by pinching up a fold of skin, which then remains as a ridge and subsides abnormally slowly. The normal loss of elasticity of the skin with age makes this an unsatisfactory sign in the elderly

(contd)

Dry mouth	Can be a sign of dehydration but is apt to be deceptive as can be due to mouth-breathing alone
Coated mouth	Mouth can appear coated due to poor mouth hygiene. However, the most common cause is oral candida infection whereby the mouth is covered with a thick white substance which when displaced reveals red, inflamed oral mucosa
Weekly weight	Measured in kg. Patient should be weighed in same type of clothes at the same time each day. Normal circadian rhythm is that people weigh most in the evening. Recent weight loss may be due to inadequate nutritional intake, malabsorption or metabolic disturbance. Recent weight gain may be due to hypothyroidism, corticosteroid treatment or fluid retention, e.g. in cardiac failure
Nausea	Assessed by patient report. The patient may describe feeling 'sick' or 'queasy', although 'feeling sick' is sometimes used as an expression of non-specific ill health. Usually associated with vomiting in gastrointestinal disease. As an isolated symptom likely to be due to depression or neurosis
Poor appetite	Subjective to define – depends on patient's norm
Dysphagia	Difficulty in swallowing. This can be a conscious difficulty in initiating a swallow, e.g. due to a painful lesion in the mouth or throat or to a neurological disorder. Sticking of food is an important symptom in oesophageal disease. When swallowing is immediately followed by a fit of coughing, this suggests a neuromuscular disturbance, particularly when fluids are swallowed
Special diet feeding	The patient has some dietary need, e.g. diabetic diet, high protein diet, renal diet, nasogastric feeding, gastrostomy feeding or total parenteral nutrition (TPN) feeding. Usually will have been assessed by the dietician
Concentrated urine	Urine is a dark yellowish brown colour and indicates that fluid intake is poor. Needs to be distinguished from the brown beer like urine passed by patients who have hepatocellular and obstructive jaundice
Odour	Normal, fresh urine should be odourless. However, concentrated urine has a peculiar odour. An ammoniacal smell is the result of bacterial decomposition commonly present in urine that has been standing for some time. A common abnormal urinary smell is a fishy smell, which is caused by infection with *Escherichia coli*
Pain on micturition	Patient reports a stinging or burning pain on passing urine

Frequency	The passage of smaller amounts of urine more often with no increase in overall volume of urine passed. Often indicative of urinary tract infection or anxiety
Incontinent	The involuntary passage of urine
Catheterized	The presence of an indwelling urinary foley catheter
Bowels open	The passage of faecal matter. Assessed by observation or patient report
Constipated stool	The stool passed is hard and difficult to pass. Usually due to a longer transit in the bowel so more water is reabsorbed resulting in hard stool. This can be caused by many factors, e.g. reduced mobility, inadequate amounts of fibre in diet, inadequate privacy for defecation, partial intestinal obstruction, spinal cord compression that affects bowel function, hypothyroidism and the effects of some pharmaceutical agents, e.g. narcotic analgesics, antidepressants
Loose stool	The stool passed is watery and not properly formed. Needs to be carefully distinguished from liquid 'overflow' stool associated with impacted stool in extreme constipation
Faecal incontinence	The involuntary passage of stool
Body temperature	Estimated in °C by placing a thermometer under the tongue, in the rectum or under the axilla (safest route for patients who are confused or have reduced consciousness, although thought to be less accurate). Rectal temperature is usually 0.5°C higher than the mouth temperature, which is in turn 0.5°C higher than the axilla temperature. Normal oral temperature is 37°C. Circadian rhythm of about 0.5°C occurs – lowest temperature being in the early morning. Therefore it is recommended to take temperature in the early evening for highest daily measurement. Any temperature of around 35°C must be checked with a subnormal range thermometer
Skin: hot	Warmth of skin to touch usually provides a remarkably good indication of fever
cool	Coolness of skin to touch gives a totally unreliable estimate of normal or low temperature (the skin of a patient with normal temperature may feel cold and an apparently normal skin temperature does not exclude hypothermia). Skin may feel cool where there is peripheral vasoconstriction, e.g. in shock, although cutaneous features are poor indicators of the shock state
Cyanotic – central	Occurs when 5gdl of haemoglobin are deoxygenated. This occurs when the blood is not properly oxygenated in the lungs, e.g. in severe heart failure, severe lung

(contd)

	disease, right to left cardiac shunt or in polycythaemia. With central cyanosis the tongue, lips and nail beds are all blue. Occurs when arterial oxygen saturation is between 80 and 85%
Cyanotic – peripheral	Occurs when the circulating blood is adequately oxygenated but a local abnormality of peripheral circulation makes one or more of the extremities appear blue. With peripheral cyanosis the nails beds are blue in colour. Common causes include cold, poor and slow blood flow due to arterial blockage or when venous return to the heart is obstructed by occlusion of a vein so the blue colour of the venous blood becomes apparent. Also occurs when cardiac output is decreased to the extent where vasoconstriction diverts blood flow from the skin
Pale	Subjective assessment of skin colour probably best judged from the face. Skin may have a colourless or transparent appearance. Can be due to vasoconstriction, e.g. in fright, shock or anaemia
Jaundice	Jaundice is obvious clinically when the total serum bilirubin rises three times the normal level (50 μmol/l; 3.0 mg/100 ml). It is best detected in the sclerae of the eyes where the bilirubin colours the elastic tissue yellow. As the jaundice deepens the skin colour may change from a lemon tinge to deep yellow and eventually to a greenish brown colour
Reddening of pressure areas	The presence of non-blanching erythaemia in a area of skin which has been the site where pressure has been exerted
Ulceration/damage	The presence of an area of skin that has been damaged so that the skin surface is broken. The resultant wound can be of various depths involving the epidermis only or all skin layers and deep facia
Purulent wound	The presence of a wound that is covered or partially covered with greenish yellow slough or exudate and usually has an unpleasant odour. The wound margin is likely to be red and inflamed
Limb: weakness/flaccid	Weakness denotes a loss of muscle power. Varies according to extent of damage, e.g. no active muscle contraction, movement which is possible with gravity eliminated, movement which is possible against gravity, movement which is possible against gravity and resistance but which is weaker than normal. Flaccidity (hypotonia) is a decreased muscle resistance or tone, although is difficult to distinguish from good relaxation
contracture/ spasticity	A contracture is a permanent restriction of extension. Hypertonia is an increased muscle resistance or tone and can be spastic or rigid. In spasticity, the resistance

	to passive movement increases initially and as the movement is continued the resistance falls away, whereas rigid hypertonia produces a resistance that feels uniform throughout the movement, although it may be jerky. Muscle tone will be difficult to examine if the patient is cold, nervous or if movement will cause or be expected to cause pain and so cause the patient to resist movement
Tingling	An example of paraesthesiae or altered sensation that occurs as a result of a disturbance in the sensory nervous system. Other sensations include 'numbness', 'tightness' or 'pins and needles'. Assessed by patient report
Visual disturbance	Assessed by patient report. Disturbances in vision include sudden blindness, double vision, blurred vision, some visual field loss or additional objects in visual field, e.g. floaters, zigzag lines and flashing lights. In some cases, the patient may not be aware of a visual problem, e.g. hemianopia post-CVA with resulting inattention
Lethargic	Excessive tiredness, 'having no energy', drowsiness. Difficult to define and is subjective. Can be a sign of various situations from lack of sleep on an open ward, to anaemia, depression or reduced consciousness in an acute neurological or cardiac event
Disorientated	There are three aspects to orientation, in place, in time and in person. A disorientated patient will give inaccurate answers to one or all of these. Disorientation is a cardinal symptom of confusional states and dementia. Recent events must be taken into account, e.g. someone who has been taken into hospital in the middle of the night may not be able to name the hospital but should be in no doubt that they are in hospital
Slurred/dysarthric	Defective speech articulation due to poorly co-ordinated movements of the lips, tongue and palate (or possibly ill-fitting dentures). Varies in severity from complete inability to articulate to very minor slurring of speech
Dysphasic	A language defect in putting thoughts into words (expressive) or understanding the spoken word (receptive)

Appendix 9
Definition of items on the Byron Physical Assessment Framework after refinement by expert group

Item on physical assessment framework	Assessment definition	Possible significance of abnormality
Respiration: rate (normal 12–18 breaths/min)	Number of full breaths, i.e. inspiration and expiration phases counted in one full minute while the patient is at rest. Should be assessed by surreptitiously observing the movement of the chest wall to avoid drawing the patient's attention to breathing, which may alter the rate	The rate is increased in a variety of pathological states, including pyrexia, acute pulmonary infections and conditions where there is a sudden increase in the work of breathing, e.g. bronchial asthma and acute pulmonary oedema. The rate may be decreased in diabetic coma, drug-induced respiratory depression and increased intracranial pressure
Laboured/breathless	Breathlessness is described as an uncomfortable awareness of the need to breathe. It is assessed by patient report, as there is no direct correlation between the observed rate of breathing and the subjective sensation of breathlessness. Laboured breathing is where the effort of breathing is increased and is assessed by observation of the patient for use of accessory muscles of respiration by which the whole thoracic cage is in effect lifted off the diaphragm with every breath. In some situations, patients may have laboured breathing without the experience of respiratory discomfort. Frequently laboured breathing and breathlessness will coincide but they are not mutually exclusive	Pathological causes include an increase in the work of breathing, e.g. airway obstruction (e.g. chronic obstructive airways disease, asthma) or restricted chest expansion; an increase in pulmonary ventilation due to an increase in the volume of respiratory dead space (e.g. pulmonary embolism); severe hypoxia (e.g. pneumonia or pulmonary oedema) or metabolic acidosis (e.g. ketoacidosis or renal failure); and weakness of the muscles of respiration (e.g. poliomyelitus). Anxiety is thought to influence the subjective feeling of breathlessness
Other abnormality	Other abnormalities of respiration are concerned with depth, pattern and symmetry of chest movement. Assessed by observation of the patient for as long as necessary to detect any abnormality. Normal respiration has a regular and even pattern. Chest wall movements are normally symmetrical	The depth of breathing may be considerably increased, e.g. in massive pulmonary embolism or diabetic acidosis, or shallow, e.g. when breathing is restricted by certain types of pulmonary disease or by pain. Cheyne-Stokes breathing is a cyclical variation in the depth of breathing, which usually indicates neurological dysfunction. In normal breathing, chest expansion should be symmetrical. Unilaterally reduced

	expansion may indicate local pathology, e.g. consolidation, pleural effusion or pneumothorax. Paradoxical inward movement of part of the rib cage during inspiration indicates a flail segment	Although a cough is a principal symptom of respiratory disease, it can occur in the absence of disease, e.g. clearing the throat or when food 'goes down the wrong way'. Therefore a cough is generally a symptom of abnormal pathology only when it occurs more than once and is involuntary. The nature, duration and sound of a cough varies: it can be productive (e.g. bronchitis) or unproductive (e.g. early stages of acute pneumonia); it can be prolonged (e.g. chronic bronchitis or chronic asthma); it can sound bubbly (e.g. with swallowing deficiency); harsh and 'croupy' (e.g. laryngitis), weak (e.g. with respiratory muscle weakness or when coughing causes pain) or 'wheezy' (e.g. acute bronchitis or acute asthma)	Appearance can be serous (clear, watery or frothy, e.g. in pulmonary oedema), mucoid (clear, grey or white, e.g. in chronic bronchitis/chronic asthma) or purulent (yellow, green or brown, e.g. in pulmonary infection). Haemoptysis is when blood is coughed up. This needs to be differentiated from haematemesis and nasopharyngeal bleeding. Haemoptysis is likely when blood definitely comes up with a cough, is mixed with or streaked in the sputum. Blood from the chest is usually bright red, not brown. Occurs in several conditions, e.g. pulmonary infarction (associated with pleuritic pain and breathlessness) and pneumonia (associated with fever, purulent sputum and signs of consolidation)
Cough		A cough involves making a forced expiratory effort against a closed glottis, which suddenly opens resulting in an explosive release of air which may carry with it respiratory secretions. The cough reflex is caused by stimuli arising in the mucosa of any part of the respiratory tract to the smaller bronchi. Assessed by patient report and direct observation to determine the frequency, nature, duration and sound of the cough. Associated symptoms should also be assessed, e.g. cyanosis, breathlessness, distress	
Sputum		Sputum is a respiratory tract secretion produced with certain abnormal conditions. Amount produced in 24 hours, appearance and duration should be determined. Assessed by patient report and direct observation. Patients may not know the term 'sputum', 'phlegm' may be better. Ideally sputum should be collected and the amount measured, otherwise patients can often give a useful guide to volume in terms of an egg cupful or cupful in 24 hours	

(contd)

Item on physical assessment framework	Assessment definition	Possible significance of abnormality
Added sounds	Added sounds are any sounds that can be heard in addition to the normal breath sounds. Should be assessed by auscultation. The patient should be asked to take some deep breaths with his or her mouth open while breath sounds are listened to using a stethoscope at various positions on the chest wall, ensuring the sound at each position is compared with the sound on the corresponding position on the opposite side of the chest (see diagram). The type and amplitude of breath sounds, the type of any added sounds, their position in the respiratory cycle and the extent to which they occur in the lung field should be assessed. Should any added sounds be heard the patient should be asked to cough. If the sounds are due to normal secretions in the airways, they will disappear or diminish after coughing. In normal breath sounds inspiratory airflow is heard as a characteristic rustling sound, which increases in intensity during inspiration but fades away soon after expiration begins Approximate sites for routine auscultation (posterior similar)	With bronchial breath sounds, both inspiratory and expiratory airflow is heard to be of equal length with a pause between the end of inspiration and the end of expiration (resembles the sound heard directly over the larynx or trachea), and occurs over areas of consolidation and collapse. Wheezes are musical sounds produced by the passage of air through narrowed airways. They are invariably louder during expiration and often confined to that part of the respiratory cycle, and are a cardinal symptom of airflow obstruction, e.g. in bronchial asthma and acute and chronic bronchitis. Wheezes are heard diffusely over both lung fields. Stridor is a loud, mainly inspiratory noise usually heard at the mouth, indicative of major airway obstruction. Crackles are intermittent, non-musical, short sounds most often due to the sudden opening of lightly occluded airways when gas passes through. Crackles caused by secretions within the large bronchi, e.g. in acute or chronic bronchitis are widespread, bilateral, audible during inspiration and alter after coughing. Crackles that are heard in the second half of inspiration and are uninfluenced by coughing are likely to be due to parenchymal lung conditions, e.g. interstitial pulmonary oedema. A pleural rub is a leathery or creaking sound produced by movement of the visceral pleura over the parietal pleura when the surfaces are inflamed. It is usually heard towards the end of inspiration and just after the beginning of expiration, is not altered by coughing and occurs in conditions with pleural inflammation, e.g. pleurisy

Blood pressure (normal 100/60–140/90 mmHg)	Arterial blood pressure (BP) is estimated in mmHg using a sphygmomanometer. Systolic BP is the point where the pulse is first heard and is the maximum arterial pressure as the aortic valve opens and left ventricle contracts. The diastolic BP is the point where the pulse disappears and is the minimum arterial pressure when the aortic valve is closed and the left ventricle is relaxing. When taking the blood pressure, the brachial pulse and the sphygmomano-meter should be on the same level as the heart	Hypotension is a sign of reduced blood volume, cardiac failure and sepsis. Hypertension is a symptom of ischaemic heart disease, peripheral vascular disease and renal disease
Heart rate: (normal 65–95 beats/min)	Generally the radial pulse is taken as a measurement of heart rate, although in some situations it may not be the same. Pulse rate value is generally assumed to denote number of heartbeats per minute and should be taken at rest. Pulse should be assessed over a minute to ensure that any irregularities and abnormalities have been assessed	Bradycardia (rate < 60) can occur in hypothyroidism, hypothermia, digoxin toxicity and complete heart block. Tachycardia (rate > 100) can occur in cardiac arrhythmias, e.g. supraventricular tachycardia and atrial flutter, sepsis, shock
irregular	The normal heart rate should be of regular, even rhythm and volume. Assessed by palpating the radial pulse for one minute (at the same time as the heart rate is assessed) and also patient report concerning the occurrence of palpitations. An irregular pulse can be regularly or irregularly irregular. Should the pulse be irregular in any way the apex beat should also be assessed for rate and rhythm and any deficit between the apex and radial beats determined	Irregularities in heart rate are usually caused by cardiac arrhythmias, e.g. a regularly irregular pulse is often due to second degree heart block and an irregularly irregular pulse is often due to atrial fibrillation. Palpitation can be described as an awareness of heartbeat. While awareness of heart-beat is normal at times of physical exertion or emotional stimulation, an awareness of heartbeat where the heart 'lurches', 'jumps out of the chest', 'misses a beat', is 'all over the place' or 'hit one, miss one' can signify the occurrence of extrasystoles. Runs of palpitations where the patient is aware of a rapid heart beat signifies cardiac arrhythmia, e.g. atrial fibrillation, and paroxysmal tachycardia

(contd)

Item on physical assessment framework	Assessment definition	Possible significance of abnormality
weak pulse	Generally the pulse is said to be weak when it is difficult to palpate, i.e. the rise and fall of the blood vessel feels faint under the finger. It is usually the radial pulse that is assessed	Systolic BP of over 50 mmHg is generally required to palpate a radial pulse and therefore the pulse feels weak in conditions where BP is low, e.g. shock, cardiac failure
Chest pain	Assessed by patient report and sometimes by observation of patient facial expression and posture. Description of the pain should be obtained, e.g. main site, radiation, character, severity, duration, frequency and periodicity, special times of occurrence, aggravating factors, relieving factors and associated phenomena	Can be due to cardiac ischaemia, where patients often describe chest pain that is 'tight', 'pressing' or 'crushing'. It frequently radiates to the left arm and less frequently to the right arm, back, neck, jaw and teeth. Important non-cardiac chest pain includes pleuritic pain (sharp, stabbing pain aggravated by breathing/coughing), musculoskeletal pain (continuous and dull ache) and heartburn (substernal burning pain often confused with cardiac pain)
Calf pain/swelling	Calf pain is assessed by patient report. Description of the pain should be obtained. Calf swelling is assessed by direct observation of both calves. If in any doubt each calf should be measured at the widest part with a tape measure	Unilateral calf pain is often caused by deep vein thrombosis (DVT). Pain occurs when the muscle mass containing the affected vein is squeezed. In the presence of a venous thrombosis of the calf, sharp dorsiflexion of the foot may be painful (Homan's sign). In the presence of a DVT, calf swelling will be unilateral. Other associated signs of DVT are warmth and discoloration of the skin, although these signs are not very reliable
Dizziness	Assessed by patient report and sometimes direct observation should a patient be observed stumbling or sitting down suddenly after standing up. Patients often describe dizziness as giddiness, floating on air, faintness or light-headedness	Common causes include anaemia, postural hypotension, dehydration, phenytoin toxicity or side effects of other drugs, e.g. oxybutinin

Pitting oedema	Occurs when fluid collects in the tissues of the feet and ankles (or sacrum if patient is lying in bed). Assessed by pressing the tissue firmly over bone. In the presence of pitting oedema, an imprint of the fingers will be left, as the fluid in the tissues is displaced and will gradually fill in when the pressure is released. Extent of oedema should be assessed and it is suggested that assessment begin at the upper surface of the feet	Oedema occurs when the venous pressure plus the hydrostatic pressure of the upright posture exceeds the oncotic pressure of the plasma. Common causes are heart failure and low plasma albumen, in which case the ankle swelling is symmetrical. In cases when ankle swelling is asymmetrical, it is likely to be due to DVT or reduced muscle tone in the weak leg as a result of a cerebrovascular accident (CVA)
Cyanotic – central	Central cyanosis is a sign of hypoxia and is assessed by observation of the tongue, lips and nail beds, which are all blue in colour when central cyanosis is present	It occurs when 5 g/dl or more of haemoglobin are deoxygenated and when arterial oxygen saturation is between 80 and 85%. This occurs when the blood is not properly oxygenated in the lungs, e.g. in severe heart failure, severe lung disease, right to left cardiac shunt or in polycythaemia
Cyanotic – peripheral	Assessed by observation of the tongue, lips and nail beds. With peripheral cyanosis the nail beds only are blue in colour	Occurs when the circulating blood is adequately oxygenated but a local abnormality of peripheral circulation makes one or more of the extremities appear blue. Common causes include the cold, poor and slow blood flow due to arterial blockage or when venous return to the heart is obstructed by occlusion of a vein so the blue colour of the venous blood becomes apparent. Also occurs when cardiac output is decreased to the extent where vasoconstriction diverts blood flow from the skin
Pale	Assessed by observation of skin colour. Probably best judged from examining the palpebral conjunctiva of the lower eyelid, although this may be reddened unduly by factors such as rubbing, hay fever, conjunctivitis or lack of sleep. The skin on the face is another useful site where it may have a colourless or transparent appearance	Pallor may be due to anaemia or vasoconstriction, e.g. in fright, clinical shock or a faint

(contd)

Item on physical assessment framework	Assessment definition	Possible significance of abnormality
Body temperature	Estimated in °C by placing a thermometer in the sublingual pockets, in the rectum or under the axilla (safest route for patients who are confused or have reduced consciousness, although thought to be less accurate). Normal oral temperature is 37°C. The correlation between oral, rectal and axilla temperature is unclear. The rectal temperature is thought to be the most accurate estimate of core temperature but is the least responsive to change. The axilla temperature on the other hand is thought to be the least accurate estimate of core temperature but is very responsive to change in temperature. Circadian rhythm of about 0.5°C occurs – lowest temperature being in the early morning. Therefore it is recommended that daily temperature readings are taken in the early evening for highest daily measurement. Any temperature of around 35.5°C must be checked with a subnormal range thermometer	Commonly fever, i.e. a temperature over 37°C, is due to infection, although there are many non-infective causes including tissue necrosis (myocardial infarction, pulmonary infarction and trauma), severe anaemia and certain types of malignancy. Hypothermia occurs with a core temperature of less than 35°C. In hypothermic patients, it is not possible to record an accurate oral or axilla temperature and therefore rectal temperature should be recorded. Common causes of hypothermia include exposure to cold, hypothyroidism, hypoglycaemia, under nutrition and any severe illness
Skin: hot	Assessed by touching the patient's cheek or forehead, which will feel hot to touch. Some patients may look flushed and/or may perspire	Warmth of skin to touch usually provides a remarkably good indication of fever
cool/clammy	Assessed by touching the patient's face, which will feel cool. Clammy skin will feel moist to touch and is often associated with pallor	Skin may feel cool and/or clammy where there is peripheral vasoconstriction, e.g. in shock, although cutaneous features are poor indicators of the shocked state. Coolness of skin to touch gives an unreliable estimate of normal or low temperature (the skin of a patient with normal temperature may feel

Weekly weight	Measured in kg. Patient should be weighed in same type of clothes at the same time each day. Normal circadian rhythm is that people weigh most in the evening. Weekly weight readings should be compared with previous readings, as identifying a pattern of weight gain or loss is often important in assessing abnormal pathology	cold and an apparently normal skin temperature does not exclude hypothermia) Recent weight loss may be due to inadequate nutritional intake, malabsorption or metabolic disturbance. Recent weight gain may be due to hypothyroidism, corticosteroid treatment or fluid retention, e.g. in cardiac failure (in which case more frequent weight recording needs to be considered)
Reduced tissue turgor	This can be assessed by gently pinching up a fold of skin just below the collarbone between thumb and forefinger. Skin should return to its normal position when released within 30 seconds	Loss of elasticity of the skin can be a sign of dehydration where the fold of skin remains as a ridge for over 30 seconds before returning to its normal position. The normal loss of elasticity of the skin with age makes this an unreliable sign in the elderly
Dry mouth	Assessed by patient report of having a dry mouth, confirmed by direct observation. Observation should be conducted with a torch. Normal buccal mucosa is greyish red and appears moist	Can be a sign of dehydration but is apt to be deceptive as can be due to mouth-breathing alone
Coated mouth	Assessed by patient report of having a sore mouth and direct observation of the mouth and throat using a torch. A coated mouth will be completely or partially covered in a substance that obscures the colour of the normal buccal mucosa and which does not disperse after drinking	Mouth can appear coated due to poor mouth hygiene. However, the most common cause is oral candida infection whereby the mouth and/or throat has patches of a thick white substance which covers red, inflamed oral mucosa
Poor appetite	Assessed by patient report and direct observation of what and how much the patient eats. Needs to be considered in light of other factors, including usual appetite and level of activity	Can be caused by gastrointestinal disease, e.g. gastric ulceration, gastric carcinoma. Other possible causes are depression, loss of taste, and unsuitable type and presentation of food

(contd)

Item on physical assessment framework	Assessment definition	Possible significance of abnormality
Nausea/vomiting	Nausea is assessed by patient report. The patient may describe feeling 'sick' or 'queasy', although 'feeling sick' is sometimes used as an expression of non-specific ill health. Usually associated with vomiting in gastrointestinal disease. Vomiting is assessed by patient report and direct observation. The frequency and timing of vomiting and appearance and amount of the vomit should be assessed	Conditions characterized by vomiting include gastric outlet obstruction where copious amounts of undigested food are vomited, ulcerative lesions of upper gastrointestinal tract where fresh or altered blood are vomited, acute gastritis and acute cholecystitis. Non-gastrointestinal causes of vomiting include labyrinthine disorders, raised intracranial pressure, severe pain, renal failure, digoxin toxicity and side effects of medications, e.g. oral potassium chloride, aminophylline and antibiotics
Abdominal pain/ distension	Abdominal pain is assessed by patient report. Onset, duration, type and circumstances of pain should be assessed. Abdominal distension is assessed by observation of the abdomen, which may also feel firm if distended	An intense, constant, generalized pain of quick onset may imply perforation of a peptic ulcer, acute pancreatitis or a ruptured aortic aneurysm; a waxing, waning pain felt over the abdomen may be due to intestinal obstruction; while an acute colicky pain associated with diarrhoea and vomiting is likely to be due to an enteric infection. Abdominal distension is commonly due to the five Fs – fat, fluid, faeces, flatus and foetus. Fluid or ascites is commonly due to liver disease, abdominal malignancy or cardiac failure. Flatus can be caused by air swallowing or high fibre diets or more serious disorders, e.g. large bowel obstruction or sigmoid volvulus. Extreme faecal impaction may cause abdominal distension
Jaundice	Assessed by observation. It is best detected in the sclerae of the eyes, where the bilirubin colours the elastic tissue a lemon-yellow colour but can be detected in the skin	Jaundice is obvious clinically when the total serum bilirubin rises to three times the normal level (50 μmol/l; 3.0 mg/ 100ml). As the jaundice deepens, the skin colour may change from a lemon tinge to deep yellow and eventually to a greenish brown colour. Assessment of skin colour is more

		difficult in patients with dark skin, and the yellow fat in the sclera of Afro-Caribbean patients may simulate jaundice
Dysphagia	Dysphagia is difficulty in swallowing and is assessed by patient report, sometimes direct observation and speech therapy reports. Patients who consistently cough after food and especially fluids may have a swallowing defect	Dysphagia can be a conscious difficulty in initiating a swallow, e.g. due to a painful lesion in the mouth or throat, or to a neurological disorder where patients may not be aware that they have impaired swallowing. Sticking of food in the oesophagus after swallowing is an important symptom in oesophageal disease. When swallowing is immediately followed by a fit of coughing, this suggests a neuromuscular disturbance resulting in possible aspiration, particularly when fluids are swallowed
Special diet feeding	Assessed by patient report if dietary need is long-standing or dietician report	The patient has some dietary need, e.g. diabetic diet, high protein diet, renal diet, nasogastric feeding, gastrostomy feeding or TPN feeding
Bowels open (yes or no)	The passage of faecal matter. Assessed by observation, patient report or report of a nursing colleague	
Hard, dry stool	Assessed by observation and patient report. Normal stool is soft, brown, formed and easy to pass. Hard, dry stool may have a pellet-like appearance	Hard, dry stool that is difficult to pass occurs in constipation and is usually due to a longer transit in the bowel during which more water is reabsorbed. This can be caused by many factors, e.g. reduced mobility, inadequate amounts of fibre in diet, inadequate privacy for defecation, partial intestinal obstruction, spinal cord compression that affects bowel function, hypothyroidism and the effects of some pharmaceutical agents, e.g. narcotic analgesics, antidepressants
Loose stool	Assessed by observation and patient report. The stool passed is watery and not properly formed	Possible causes of loose stool include irritable bowel syndrome, gastrointestinal irritation due to infection, e.g.

(contd)

Item on physical assessment framework	Assessment definition	Possible significance of abnormality
		Clostridium difficile, and side effects of drugs, e.g. antibiotics. Melaena, the black, tarry stool passed as a result of upper gastrointestinal bleeding, is usually loose. A careful distinction needs to be made between loose stool and the liquid 'overflow' stool associated with impacted stool in extreme constipation
Faecal incontinence	Assessed by observation or patient report. It is the involuntary passage of stool. Also includes the need for manual evacuation of faeces	Common causes include neurological dysfunction, e.g. multiple sclerosis and dementia. Faecal incontinence in the absence of urinary incontinence is usually caused by local bowel pathology, which includes faecal impaction, acute infective diarrhoea, colonic tumours, diverticular disease and inflammatory bowel disease
Other abnormality	Other abnormalities of bowel function include abnormal appearance, smell or consistency of stool, pain on passing stool and alteration of normal bowel habit. Assessed by observation and patient report. Normal bowel pattern varies between several evacuations per day to one every three days, and normal stool is brown in colour, formed, soft and easy to pass	Changes in habit may signify underlying disease, e.g. irritable bowel disease or side effects of prescribed medications. Stool may appear black, e.g. upper GI bleed or if patient is taking oral iron; tarry black with a distinctive offensive smell (meleena), e.g. severe upper GI bleed; pale, bulky and particularly offensive (steatorrhoea), e.g. in small bowel malabsorption; mixed with blood and mucus, e.g. inflammatory bowel disease. Liquid 'overflow' stool can have a particularly offensive smell. Bleeding per rectum can be caused by haemorrhoids, inflammatory bowel disease and diverticular disease. Pain on passing stool may be caused by haemorrhoids or constipation
Dysuria	Strictly speaking the term dysuria means difficulty passing urine, although it is commonly used to	Pain on passing urine usually indicates the presence of a urinary tract infection, which is precipitated by many factors

	denote pain on micturition. Assessed by patient report of a stinging or burning pain on passing urine, of difficulty initiating the passing of urine or of poor stream	including poor fluid intake and incomplete bladder emptying. Difficulty in passing urine occurs more commonly in men, due to prostate hypertrophy, and is characterized by hesitancy, poor tream and post-micturition dribbling. Urinary s retention can occur due to neurological deficits or can be drug induced, e.g. pethidine
Frequency/urgency	Assessed by patient report and observation. Frequency is the passage of smaller amounts of urine more often with no increase in overall volume of urine passed. Most people pass urine 3–6 times during the day and passing urine 7 times or more a day is considered abnormally high. Generally it is unusual to be woken at night to pass urine, although some people always have to get up once during the night. Being woken twice or more is considered abnormal frequency, although in the very elderly this is commonplace as the normal diurnal variation in urinary excretion is lost. Urgency is the strong desire to pass urine, which may be followed by incontinence if the opportunity to void is not available	Both frequency and urgency are indicative of urinary tract infection, detrusor muscle instability, prostatic enlargement, diuretic treatment or anxiety
Concentrated urine	Assessed by direct observation or sometimes patient report. Concentrated urine is a dark yellowish brown colour	Indicates that the patient is dehydrated
Odour	Assessed by direct observation. Normal, fresh urine should be odourless	Concentrated urine has a peculiar odour. An ammoniacal smell is the result of bacterial decomposition commonly present in urine that has been standing for some time. A common abnormal urinary smell is a fishy smell, which is caused by infection with *Escherichia coli*

(contd)

Item on physical assessment framework	Assessment definition	Possible significance of abnormality
Incontinent	Assessed by observation and patient report. Incontinence is the involuntary passage of urine	This can involve the passage of small amounts of urine on laughing, coughing or lifting in women, especially those who have had children and have weak pelvic floor muscles. In men, post-micturition dribbling can occur, e.g. in urethral obstruction such as prostate hypertrophy. Other causes of incontinence include neurological disturbance of bladder function, constipation, dementia and difficulty getting to the toilet or arranging clothing
Catheterized	Assessed by observation and patient report. Denotes the presence of an indwelling urinary foley catheter (urethral or supra-pubic) or the use of intermittent self-catheterization	Patients are catheterized when accurate measurement of urinary output is necessary, for acute or chronic retention of urine or in selected situations for the management of incontinence after full investigation and trial of other available treatments
Headache	Assessed by patient report. Description of the pain should be obtained, i.e. location, radiation, character, severity, duration, frequency and periodicity, special times of occurrence, aggravating factors, relieving factors and associated phenomena	Common causes of recurrent or persistent headache include tension headaches, migraine and cranial arteritus (in the elderly). Less common causes include raised intracranial pressure and hypertension, which, although frequently blamed, is not often the cause. The typical hypertension headache is worse on waking, occipital in site and pounding in character
Visual disturbance	Assessed by patient report and observation of patient's functional ability. Disturbances in vision include sudden blindness, double vision, blurred vision, some visual field loss, isolated visual hallucinations or additional objects in visual field, e.g. floaters, zigzag lines and flashing lights	Can occur when there is damage to the nervous system, e.g. in CVA, or due to interruption to the blood flow to the eye, e.g. in retinal artery or retinal vein thrombosis or cranial arteritis. In some cases, the patient may not be aware of a visual problem, e.g. hemianopia post-CVA with resulting inattention

Paraesthesiae	Assessed by patient report of any altered sensation, e.g. the experience of 'tingling', 'numbness', 'pins and needles' or 'tightness'. Description of location, severity and duration should be obtained	Generally occurs as a result of a disturbance in the sensory nervous system. Over-breathing due to fright or anxiety may cause 'pins and needles' around the mouth and in the fingers
Lethargic/mood change	Assessed by patient report and observation during normal daily interaction. Lethargy can be described as excessive tiredness, 'having no energy' and drowsiness. Mood change is when the patient's mood state changes. Mood states include happy, sad, dejected, miserable, depressed, anxious, panic stricken, ecstatic, suspicious, perplexed and so on. Discussion with relatives may be helpful for further assessment	Lethargy can be a sign of various situations from lack of sleep on an open ward, to anaemia, depression or reduced consciousness in an acute neurological or cardiac event. Marked mood change may be found in organic brain disease, metabolic disorders, e.g. thyroid over activity/deficiency, drug reaction or acute psychiatric disorder
Disorientated/confused	Assessed by observation of and normal interaction with the patient. There are three aspects to orient-ation: in place, in time and in person. A disorientated patient will give inaccurate answers to one or all of these. Recent events must be taken into account, e.g. someone who has been taken into hospital in the middle of the night may not be able to name the hospital but should be in no doubt that they are in hospital. Confusion and cognitive impairment may involve disorientation, inappropriate actions and speech, decreased level of awareness, memory impairment, delusions, altered attention and restlessness	Disorientation is a cardinal symptom of confusional states and dementia. Confusional states, particularly in the elderly, are common non-specific presentations of almost any disorder, physical or mental. If confusion is acute and of sudden onset then a physical cause is more likely, e.g. infection, heart failure or medication induced. A gradual and lengthy onset may be due to dementia and if linked to major life event, e.g. a bereavement or sudden change of surroundings, may signify a depressive state, which can present as confusion in the elderly. A mini-mental state examination may be of use for further assessments
Slurred speech/dysarthric	Assessed by observation of a patient's speech during normal interaction. Dysarthria is defective speech articulation due to poorly co-ordinated	Usually occurs as a result of neurological damage, e.g. CVA, Parkinson's disease or weakness of the articulating muscles due to myopathy. A cleft palate will cause slurred speech, as

(contd)

Item on physical assessment framework	Assessment definition	Possible significance of abnormality
	movements of the lips, tongue and palate. Varies in severity from complete inability to articulate to very minor slurring of speech	will ill-fitting dentures
Dysphasic	Assessed by observation during normal daily interaction and at times patient report. Dysphasia is a language defect in putting thoughts into words (expressive) or understanding the spoken word (receptive), although it is usually a combination of both. In expressive dysphasia, patients are able to comprehend language satisfactorily, know what they want to say but are unable to say it. Vocabulary is reduced and errors in pronunciation and grammar are common. Can be further assessed by asking patients to name objects. In receptive dysphasia, comprehension of speech is impaired and is always accompanied by derangement of the patient's use of language. Although pronunciation and fluency may be normal, much of the patient's speech is irrelevant in content. Can be further assessed by asking the patient to do things, e.g. 'hold out your hand'. Assessment should differentiate dysphasia from deafness. Accurate assessment may be difficult where English is not first language	Occurs as a result of neurological damage, most commonly in CVAs
Limb: weakness/flaccid	Assessed by observation and at times patient report. Weakness denotes a loss of muscle power. Can be observed as patient conducts functional activities, e.g. walking, dressing, or by purposeful	Causes of muscle weakness include neurological damage, e.g. CVA, multiple sclerosis, and as a result of generalized loss of muscle tissue associated with some systemic or metabolic disease

	examination, e.g. asking the patient to squeeze both the examiner's hands with theirs, lift their arms over their head, lift their legs off the surface of the bed while lying down. Muscle power of both legs and of both arms should be compared. Muscle power varies according to extent of damage and can be further categorized, e.g. no active muscle contraction, movement which is possible with gravity eliminated, movement which is possible against gravity, movement which is possible against gravity and resistance but which is weaker than normal. Flaccidity (hypotonia) is a decreased muscle resistance or tone, although it is difficult to distinguish from good relaxation	
contracture/stiffness	Assessed by observing joint movement during normal daily activities. Also by patient report of stiffness. Can be further assessed by moving joints through their range of movement and observing any limitations. A contracture is a permanent restriction of joint movement as a result of prolonged immobilization of the joint in one position, which causes muscle fibres to shorten and atrophy to occur. Hypertonia is an increased muscle resistance or tone and can be spastic or rigid. In spasticity, the resistance to passive movement increases initially and as the movement is continued, the resistance falls away, whereas rigid hypertonia produces a resistance that feels uniform throughout the movement, although it may be jerky. Muscle tone will be difficult to examine if the patient is	Contractures may result in any situation where the patient is immobile for a length of time. Spasticity results from upper motor neurone damage and rigidity occurs in diseases of the basal ganglia

(contd)

Item on physical assessment framework	Assessment definition	Possible significance of abnormality
	cold, nervous or if movement will cause or be expected to cause pain and so cause the patient to resist movement	
Joint/muscular pain	Assessed mainly by patient report but sometimes by observing patient's posture, the way they carry out functional activities or when moving patients who need assistance to move. Assessment of pain should obtain information about main site of pain, radiation, character, severity, duration, frequency and periodicity, special times of occurrence, e.g. after a fall or injury, aggravating factors and relieving factors	Joint pain may be caused by injury, e.g. sprained ligaments, fractures; degenerative disease, e.g. rheumatoid arthritis, osteoarthritis; acute joint infection; or after periods of misuse, e.g. patients on bed rest. Muscular pain can result from joint damage, muscle sprain and bruising or from referred pain in neurological damage, e.g. sciatica
Joint/tissue swelling	Assessed by observation of joints and skin. Can be useful to compare with corresponding joint for degree of swelling	Joint swelling can be caused by injury or by degenerative disease. Tissue swelling can be caused by underlying joint or bone damage, causing localized oedema. Other causes of tissue swelling include non-pitting oedema, e.g. in lymphoedema, reduced plasma albumen
Rash	Assessed by observation of the skin. Typically is red, blotchy and can be raised above the skin surface. Can occur on any part of the body and may be itchy	Can occur as a result of dermatological condition, e.g. excema, psoriasis; as a sign of connective tissue disorders, e.g. scleroderma or systemic lupus erythematosus; as a result of an allergy, e.g. a drug reaction (e.g. antibiotics) or a food allergy (e.g. shellfish allergy is common) or an allergy to toiletries, cosmetics or washing powder; or as a result of maceration of the skin due to excessive sweating or inadequate drying

Reddening of pressure areas	Assessed by observation of areas of skin where pressure has been exerted, e.g. sacrum, hips, shoulders, heels, which are judged to be red in the presence of non-blanching erythaema. This is present when reddened skin is pressed lightly with the fingers and does not become white	This indicates that permanent damage has occurred to the micro-circulation
Skin ulceration/damage	Assessed by direct observation of an area of skin that has been damaged so that the skin surface is broken	The resultant wound can be of various depths, involving the epidermis only or all skin layers and deep facia. Can be caused by sustained pressure to the skin, disturbance to the circulation, trauma or surgically
Purulent wound	Assessed by direct observation of a wound that is covered or partially covered with greenish yellow slough or exudate, and may have an unpleasant odour. The wound margin is likely to be red and inflamed. May be associated with pyrexia	All wounds have potential to become infected. Infection may be precipitated by many factors, e.g. contamination from urine/faeces, cross-infection by hospital staff, poor patient nutrition, systemic disease or introduced prior to skin closure during surgery

Ruth Harris (1995)

References

Aggleton PJ, Chalmers HA (1986) Nursing Models and the Nursing Process. Basingstoke: MacMillan.

Algase DL, Beel-Bates CA (1993) Everyday indicators of impaired cognition: development of a new screening scale. Research in Nursing and Health 16: 57–66.

Altman DG (1991) Practical Statistics for Medical Research. London: Chapman and Hall.

Audit Commission (1992) Lying in Wait: the use of medical beds in acute hospitals. London: HMSO.

Barker P (1987) Assembling the pieces. Nursing Times 83(47): 67–68.

Batehup L, Evans A (1992) A new strategy. Nursing Times 88(47): 40–41.

Bates B (1995) A Pocket Guide to Physical Examination and History Taking, 2nd edn. Philadelphia, PA: JB Lippincott.

Beck WC, Campbell R (1975) Clinical thermometry. Guthrie Bulletin 43: 175–194.

Benner P (1984) From Novice to Expert: excellence and power in clinical nursing practice. Menlo Park: Addison-Wesley.

Bland JM, Altman DG (1986) Statistical methods for assessing agreement between two methods of clinical measurement. Lancet February 8: 307–310.

Blaylock A, Cason CL (1992) Discharge planning: predicting patients needs. Journal of Gerontological Nursing 18(7): 5–10.

Brennan P, Silman A (1992) Statistical methods for assessing observer variability in clinical measures. British Medical Journal 304: 1491.

Brians LK, Alexander K, Grota P, Chen RWH, Dumas V (1991) The development of the RISK tool for fall prevention. Rehabilitation Nursing 16(2): 67–69.

Burns C (1991) Parallels between research and diagnosis: the reliability and validity issues of clinical practice. Nurse Practitioner 16(10): 42–50.

Carboni JT (1992) Instrument development and the measurement of unitary constructs. Nursing Science Quarterly 5(3): 134–142.

Carmines EG, Zeller RA (1979) Reliability and validity assessment. Sage University Paper series on quantitative applications in the social sciences, series no 07 017. Beverly Hills and London: Sage Publications.

Chang B, Gonzales E, Caswell D (1988) Validity and reliability of an assessment guide for identifying nursing diagnoses. Australian Journal of Advanced Nursing 5(2): 16–22.

139

Choi SC, Boxerman SB, Steinburg I (1978) Nurses preference of terminal digits in data reading. Journal of Nursing Education 17(9): 38–41.

Closs J (1987) Oral temperature measurement. Nursing Times January 7: 36–39.

Cohen J (1960) A coefficient of agreement for nominal scales. Educational and Psychological Measurement 20: 37–46.

Coles MC, Fullenwider SD (1988) Managing the dilemma. Nursing Management 19(12): 65–66, 70, 72.

Conceicao S, Ward MK, Kerr DNS (1976) Defects in sphygmomanometers: an important source of error in blood pressure recording. British Medical Journal ii: 886–888.

Corcoran S (1986) Task complexity and nursing expertise as factors in decision making. Nursing Research 35 (2): 107–112.

Crandall B, Getchell-Reiter K (1993) Critical decision making: a technique for eliciting concrete assessment indicators from the intuition of NICU nurses. Advanced Nursing Science 16(1): 42–51.

Crosby L, Parsons C (1989) Clinical neurologic assessment tool: development and testing of an instrument to index neurologic status. Heart and Lung 18(2): 121–129.

Davis GC (1989) Measurement of the chronic pain experience: development of an instrument. Research in Nursing and Health 12: 221–227.

de la Cuesta C (1983) The nursing process: from development to implementation. Journal of Advanced Nursing 8: 365–371.

Elstein AS, Bordage G (1988) Psychology of clinical reasoning. In Dowie J, Elstein A (eds) Professional Judgement: a reader in clinical decision making. Cambridge, MA: University Press.

Erickson R. (1980) Oral temperature differences in relation to thermometer and technique. Nursing Research 29(3): 157–164.

Evans A, Griffiths P (1994) The Development of a Nursing-led Inpatient Service. London: King's Fund Centre.

Faucett J, Ellis V, Underwood P, Naqvi A, Wilson D (1990) The effect of Orem's self-care model on nursing care in a nursing home setting. Journal of Advanced Nursing 15: 659–666.

Fielding K, Rowley G (1990) Reliability of assessments by skilled observers using the Glasgow Coma Scale. Australian Journal of Advanced Nursing 7(4): 13–17.

Ford P, Walsh M (1994) New Rituals for Old: nursing through the looking glass. Oxford: Butterworth-Heinemann.

Forster B, Adler DC, Davis M (1970) Duration of effects of drinking iced water on temperature. Nursing Research 19: 169–170.

Fox DJ (1982) Fundamentals of Research in Nursing, 4th edn. New York: Appleton Century-Crofts.

Fulbrook P (1993) Core temperature measurement in adults: a literature review. Journal of Advanced Nursing 18: 1451–1460.

Griffiths P, Evans A (1995) Evaluation of a Nursing-led In-patient Service: an interim report. London: King's Fund Centre.

Hamers JPH, Huijer Abu-Saad H, Halfens RJG (1994) Diagnostic process and decision making in nursing: a literature review. Journal of Professional Nursing 10(3): 154–163.

Harris R (1995) An evaluation of the reliability and validity of a physical assessment framework used on a nurse-led ward. Unpublished MSc thesis, King's College, University of London.

Hayes PC, MacWalter RS (1992) Aids to Clinical Examination, 2nd edn. Edinburgh: Churchill Livingstone.

Henderson V (1966) The Nature of Nursing. London: Collier-MacMillan.

Herbert R (1989) Clinical observation. In Macleod Clark J, Hockey L, Further Research for Nursing: a new guide for the enquiring nurse. London: Scutari Press.

Holden RJ (1990) Models, muddles and medicine. International Journal of Nursing Studies 27: 223–234.

Holmes S, Mountain E (1993) Assessment of oral status: evaluation of three oral assessment guides. Journal of Clinical Nursing 2: 35–40.

Hurley AC, Volicer BJ, Hanrahan PA, Houde S, Volicer L (1992) Assessment of discomfort in advanced Alzheimer patients. Research in Nursing and Health 15: 369–377.

Hurst K, Dean A, Trickey S (1991) The recognition and non-recognition of problem-solving stages in nursing practice. Journal of Advanced Nursing 16: 1444–1455.

Iyer PW, Camp NH (1995) Nursing Documentation: a nursing process approach, 2nd edn. St Louis, MO: Mosby.

Jacobson SF (1992) Evaluating instruments for use in clinical nursing research. In Frank-Stromborg M (ed) Instruments for Clinical Nursing Research. Boston, MA: Jones and Bartlett.

Kitson A (1987) Raising standards of clinical practice: the fundamental issue of effective nursing practice. Journal of Advanced Nursing 12: 321–329.

Knapp TR (1985) Validity, reliability and neither. Nursing Research 34(3): 189.

Kratz CR (ed) (1979) The Nursing Process. London: Baillière Tindall.

Kristensen BO (1982) Which arm to measure blood pressure. Scand (suppl.): 69–73.

Landis JR, Koch GG (1977) The measurement of observer agreement for categorical data. Biometrics 33: 159–174.

Lee RE, Atkins E (1972) Spurious fever. American Journal of Nursing 72: 1094–1095.

Lewis T (1988) Leaping the chasm between nursing theory and practice. Journal of Advanced Nursing 13: 345–351.

Majesky SJ, Brester MH, Nishio KT (1978) Development of a research tool: patient indicators of nursing care. Nursing Research 27(6): 365–371.

Mallick MJ (1981) Patient assessment-based on data, not intuition. Nursing Outlook October: 600–605.

Marks-Maran D (1983) Can nurses diagnose? Nursing Times 79(4): 68–69.

Marriner A (1979) The Nursing Process: a scientific approach to nursing care, 2nd edn. St Louis, MO: Mosby.

Mayer GG, Buckley RF, Storrie KV, Zehner C, Wann M, Braden C, Vestil RM, White TL (1989) Measuring the requirements for nursing care in the acute head trauma patient. Rehabilitation Nursing 14(3): 123–126.

Mayers MG (1978) A Systematic Approach to the Nursing Care Plan, 2nd edn. New York: Appleton-Century-Crofts.

McDowell I, Newell C (1987) Measuring Health: a guide to rating scales and questionnaires. New York: Oxford University Press.

McFarlane of Llandaff, Castledine G (1982) A Guide to the Practice of Nursing Using the Nursing Process. London: Mosby.

McMillan SC, Williams FA (1989) Validity and reliability of the Constipation Assessment Scale. Cancer Nursing 12 (3): 183–188.

McMillan SC, Williams FA, Chatfield R, Camp LD (1988) A validity and reliability study of two tools for assessing and managing cancer pain. Oncology Nursing Forum 15(6): 735–741.

Millar-Craig MW, Bishop CN, Raftery EB (1978) Circadian variation on blood pressure. Lancet i: 795–797.

Miller J (1990) Assessing urinary incontinence. Journal of Gerontological Nursing 16(3): 15–19.

Mitchell PL, Parlin RW, Blackburn H (1964) Effect of vertical displacement of the arm on indirect blood pressure measurement. New England Journal of Medicine 271: 72–74.

Mulhearn S (1989) The nursing process: improving psychiatric admission assessment? Journal of Advanced Nursing 14: 808–814.

Munro J, Edwards C (1990) Macleod's Clinical Examination. Edinburgh: Churchill Livingstone.

Murphy MF, Moller MD (1993) Relapse management in neurobiological disorders: the Moller-Murphy Symptom Management Assessment Tool. Archives of Psychiatric Nursing 7(4): 226–235.

Nichols GA, Verhonick PJ (1968) Placement times for oral thermometers: a nursing study replication. Nursing Research 17: 159–161.

Nightingale FN (1859) Notes on Nursing: what it is and what it is not. London: Harrison (reissued Blackie 1974).

Nokes KM, Wheeler K, Kendrew J (1994) Development of an HIV assessment tool. IMAGE: Journal of Nursing Scholarship 26(2): 133–138.

Nunnally JC (1978) Psychometric Theory, 2nd edn. New York: McGraw-Hill.

Nursing Process Evaluation Working Group (1986) Report of the Nursing Process Evaluation Working Group. London: DHSS.

O'Brien ET, O'Malley K (1979) ABC of blood pressure measurement: observer. British Medical Journal ii: 775–776.

Orem DE (1991) Nursing: concepts of practice, 4th edn. St Louis, MO: Mosby Year Book.

Pank P (1994) An exploratory study to examine the patient assessment undertaken by nurses. Unpublished MSc thesis, King's College, University of London.

Pearson A, Vaughan B (1986) Nursing Models for Practice. Oxford: Heinemann Nursing.

Petrucci KE, Jacox A, McCormack K, Parks P, Kjerulff K, Baldwin B, Petrucci P (1992) Evaluating the appropriateness of a nurse expert system's patient assessment. Computers in Nursing 10 (6): 243–249.

Pinholt EM, Kroenke K, Hanley J, Kussman MJ, Twyman PL, Carpenter JL (1987) Functional assessment of the elderly: a comparison of standard instruments with clinical judgement. Archives of International Medicine 147, 484–488.

Polit DF, Hungler BP (1987) Nursing Research: principles and methods, 3rd edn. Philadelphia, PA: Lippincott.

Reed J, Bond S (1991) Nurses' assessment of elderly patients in hospital. International Journal of Nursing Studies 28(1): 55–64.

Reed J, Watson D (1994) The impact of the medical model on nursing practice and assessment. International Journal of Nursing Studies 31(1): 57–66.

Reed J (1989) All dressed up and nowhere to go: nursing assessment in care of the elderly. Unpublished PhD thesis, CNAA. Newcastle Polytechnic, Newcastle upon Tyne.

Riehl JP, Roy C (eds) (1980) Conceptual Models for Nursing Practice. New York: Appleton-Century-Crofts.

Rogers M (1970) An introduction to the theoretical basis of nursing. Philadelphia PA: Davis.

Roper N, Logan W, Tierney A (1980) The Elements of Nursing. Edinburgh: Churchill Livingstone.

Roy C (1980) The Roy Adaptation Model. In Conceptual Models for Nursing Practice. New York: Appleton-Century-Croft.

Siegrist L, Dettor R, Stocks B (1985) The PIE System: complete planning and documentation of nursing care. Quality Review Bulletin 189: 186.

Sigma Theta Tau International (1987) Directory of Nurse Researchers (2nd Ed.) Indianapolis. Cited in Algase DL, Beel-Bates CA (1993) Everyday indicators of impaired cognition: development of a new screening scale. Research in Nursing and Health 16: 57–66.

Tanner CA (1982) Instruction in the diagnostic process: an experimental study. In Kim MJ, Moritz D (eds) Classification of Nursing Diagnosis: proceedings of the third and fourth national conference, pp 145–152. New York: McGraw-Hill.

Tanner CA, Padrick KP, Westfall UE, Putzier DJ (1987) Diagnostic reasoning strategies of nurses and nursing students. Nursing Research 36(6): 358–363.

Tettero I, Jackson S, Wilson S (1993) Theory to practice: developing a Rogerian-based assessment tool. Journal of Advanced Nursing 18: 776–782.

Thompson DR (1981) Recording patients blood pressure: a review. Journal of Advanced Nursing 6: 283–290.

Tierney A (1984) The first step of the nursing process: assessment. In A Systematic Approach to Nursing Care: an introduction. Milton Keynes: Open University Press.

Toghill PJ (ed) (1995) Examining Patients: an introduction to clinical medicine, 2nd edn. London: Edward Arnold.

Topf M (1986) Three estimates of interrater reliability for nominal data. Nursing Research 35(4): 253–255.

Turner R, Blackwood R (1991) Lecture Notes on History Taking and Examination, 2nd edn. Oxford: Blackwell Scientific.

United Kingdom Central Council for Nursing, Midwifery and Health Visiting (UKCC) (1992) The Scope of Professional Practice. London: UKCC.

Walsh M, Ford P (1989) Nursing Rituals: research and rational actions. Oxford: Heinemann Nursing.

Walsh M (1990) From model to care plan. In Kershaw B, Salvage J (eds) Models for Nursing 2. London: John Wiley.

Walsh M (1991) Nursing Models in Clinical Practice: the way forward. London: Baillère Tindall.

Waltz CF, Strickland OL , Lenz ER (1991) Measurement in Nursing Research, 2nd edn. Philadelphia, PA: FA Davis.

Watson R (1994) Measuring feeding difficulty in patients with dementia: developing a scale. Journal of Advanced Nursing 19: 257–263.

Western Consortium for Cancer Nursing Research (1991) Development of a staging system for chemotherapy-induced stomatitus. Cancer Nursing 14(1): 6–12.

Wright S (1986) Developing and using a nursing model. In Kershaw B, Salvage J (eds) Models for Nursing. London: John Wiley.

Wright SG (1990) Building and Using a Model of Nursing, 2nd edn. London: Edward Arnold.

Index

abdominal pain/distension, BPAF definition, after refinement 128

abnormalities, action on detection of new abnormality 80–1

added sounds (respiration), BPAF definition, after refinement 122

admission, v. assessment 2

Affect Balance Scale (ABS) 17

Alzheimer's disease, discomfort assessment tool 9

appetite, poor, BPAF definition
before refinement 114
after refinement 127

assessment
activities of 1–2
v. admission 2
as basis for nursing intervention 2
BPAF as part of 22
description xv, 1–2
documentation 83
v. information collection and review 2
nurse-patient relationship and 2
an on-going activity 2
in practice 2–3
v. problem identification 2
process 83
as routine 2–3
structured v. unstructured 5
theoretical description 1–2
see also Byron Physical Assessment Framework; physical assessment

assessment tools 1–18
conceptual basis 7–8
conclusion 17–18
development methods 8–9

influence of experts 8–9
literature search 5–6
psychometric characteristics 9–17
error, random/systematic 10
purpose of 6–7
reliability 10–13
as equivalence 11–12
inter-rater reliability 11–12
as internal consistency 12–13
parallel forms reliability testing 11
as stability 10–11
test-retest reliability 10–11
rigour of 84
use of 5
validity 13–17
concurrent validity 14
construct validity 15–17
content validity 14
convergent validity 16, 17
criterion-related validity 14–15
definition 13
divergent validity 17
face validity 14
predictive validity 14–15

blood pressure
affecting inter-rater reliability 77
BPAF definition, after refinement 123

body temperature
affecting inter-rater reliability 77
BPAF definition
before refinement 115
after refinement 126

bowel function abnormalities, BPAF definition, after refinement 130

bowels open, BPAF definition
  before refinement 115
  after refinement 129
BPAF, see Byron Physical Assessment
    Framework; Byron Physical
    Assessment Framework study
Bradburn Affect Balance Scale (ABS) 17
bradycardia 123
breathing, see respiration
breathlessness, BPAF definition, after refine-
    ment 120
Byron Physical Assessment Framework
    (BPAF)
  background xv–xvi
  changes made 32–7
    content 35–6
    expert group 31–2
    in item definitions 36–7
    revised structure 33–4
    structure 32–5
  circulation section (original) 25
  circumstances of use 21
    daily assessment of patients 21, 22
    screening for transfer to the NLIU 21
  conceptual basis 22
  description 23
  development 24–6
  first version 93–4
  flow sheet format 24, 32
  history 20–1
  item definitions
    changes in 36–7
    before refinement 111–17
    after refinement 119–37
    see also individual BPAF items
  limitations 82
  and medical model 22
  oxygenation section 23
  as part of nursing assessment 22
  purpose of 21–2
  refinement of 28–32
    expert group 31–2
    literature review 28–31
  respiration section (original) 25
  as safety net 22
  second version 38, 91–2
  strengths 81
Byron Physical Assessment Framework
    (BPAF) study

aims xi, xvi
discussion 73–86
  conclusion 85
  content validity of the BPAF 79
  findings relating to previous literature
    82–4
  further research 86
  limitations of study 84–5
  limitations of the BPAF 82
  reliability of the BPAF 73–8
  strengths of the BPAF 81
  utilization of the BPAF 79–81
objectives 19
phases of xi–xiii
preliminary investigation aim 26
reliability evaluation, see reliability of the
    BPAF
utilization of the BPAF, see utilization of
    the BPAF
validity evaluation, see content validity of
    the BPAF

calf pain/swelling, BPAF definition
  before refinement 113
  after refinement 124
cardiovascular system
  abnormal physiological signs and
    symptoms, literature review 95–7
  physical assessment 88
care models
  effect on care delivery 83–4
  need for 3–4
  see also nursing models
catheterized, BPAF definition
  before refinement 115
  after refinement 132
central nervous system
  physical assessment 90
  see also neurological system
chest pain, BPAF definition
  before refinement 113
  after refinement 124
Cheyne-Stokes breathing 120
circulation section (original), of the BPAF 25
clinical expertise 82
coated mouth, BPAF definition
  before refinement 114
  after refinement 127
cognition, Everyday Indication of Impaired
    Cognition (EIIC) scale 17

concentrated urine, BPAF definition
    before refinement 114
    after refinement 131
concurrent validity 14
confusion, BPAF definition, after refinement
    133
consistency, internal, of assessment tools
    Cronbach coefficient alpha 13
    reliability as 12–13
    split-half technique 13
constipated stool, BPAF definition, before
    refinement 115
constipation assessment scale 7, 16
construct validity, of assessment tools 15–17
    concurrent validity 14
    convergent validity 16, 17
    discriminality 16, 17
    factor analysis 16, 17
    multitrait-multimethod matrix method 16
    Pain Flow Sheet (PFS) 17
    predictive validity 14–15
content validity, of assessment tools 14
content validity of the BPAF, evaluation
    study 65–71
    aims and objectives 66–71
    approach taken 65–6
    consistency of completion
        findings 68–9
        method 67–8
    discussion 79
    patient documentation and evidence of
        action
        findings 69–71
        method 69
    process of refining the BPAF 66–7
        expert opinion 66, 67
        literature review 66–7
    summary 71
contracture, BPAF definition
    before refinement 116
    after refinement 135–6
convergent validity 16, 17
cough, BPAF definition
    before refinement 112
    after refinement 121
crackles, BPAF definition
    before refinement 112

after refinement 122
criterion-related validity, of assessment tools
    14–15
    of the BPAF 65
Cronbach coefficient alpha 13
cure philosophy 3, 4
cyanosis, BPAF definitions
    central cyanosis
        before refinement 115–16
        after refinement 125
    peripheral cyanosis
        before refinement 116
        after refinement 125

dementia patients, feeding problems, assess-
    ment tool 7
diet, see special diet feeding
discharge needs of older patients, assessment
    tool 7
discriminality 16, 17
disorientation, BPAF definition
    before refinement 117
    after refinement 133
distension, abdominal, BPAF definition, after
    refinement 128
divergent validity 17
dizziness, BPAF definition
    before refinement 113
    after refinement 124
documentation, of patient assessment 83
dry mouth, BPAF definition
    before refinement 114
    after refinement 127
dysarthria, BPAF definition
    before refinement 117
    after refinement 133–4
dysphagia, BPAF definition
    before refinement 114
    after refinement 129
dysphasia, BPAF definition
    before refinement 117
    after refinement 134
dysuria, BPAF definition, after refinement
    130–1

equivalence, reliability as 11–12
Everyday Indication of Impaired Cognition
    (EIIC) scale 17

face validity, of assessment tools 14
    of the BPAF 65
factor analysis 16, 17
faecal incontinence, BPAF definition
    before refinement 115
    after refinement 130
feeding, *see* special diet feeding
flaccidity of limbs, BPAF definition
    before refinement 116
    after refinement 134–5
frequency, BPAF definition
    before refinement 115
    after refinement 131

gastrointestinal system
    abnormal   physiological   signs   and
        symptoms, literature review 103–5
    physical assessment 89
genitourinary system
    abnormal   physiological   signs   and
        symptoms, literature review 107–9
    physical assessment 89

haemoptysis 121
headache, BPAF definition, after refinement
    132
heart rate
    affecting inter-rater reliability 77–8
    BPAF definitions
        after refinement 123–4
        see also pulse rate
hypertension, *see* blood pressure
hypertonia
    BPAF definition
        before refinement 116–17
        after refinement 135–6
hypotension, *see* blood pressure
hypothermia, causes 126
hypotonia, *see* flaccidity

incontinence, BPAF definitions
    faecal
        before refinement 115
        after refinement 130
    urinary
        before refinement 115
        after refinement 132
incontinence monitoring record 6
inter-rater reliability 11–12

BPAF study
    of the BPAF as a whole 59–62, 78
    discussion, factors affecting reliability
        74–5, 76–8
    experienced assessors on acute wards
        54–5
    experienced v. novice assessor 55–9
    independent assessors on NLIU 48–50
    stability over time 43, 50–4
    summary 62–3
    definition 11
    see also reliability of the BPAF

jaundice, BPAF definition
    before refinement 116
    after refinement 128–9
joint pain, BPAF definition, after refinement
    136
joint swelling, BPAF definition, after refine-
    ment 136

laboured breathing, BPAF definition, after
    refinement 120
lethargy, BPAF definition
    before refinement 117
    after refinement 133
limbs, weaknesses of, BPAF definitions
    before refinement 116–17
    after refinement 134–5
Lying in Wait (Audit Commission Report)
    20

medical stability xv, 20
Memory-Orientation-Concentration (MOC)
    test 17
micturition, pain on, BPAF definition
    before refinement 114
    after refinement 130–1
Mini Mental Status Examination (MMSE)
    17
models of care, *see* care models; nursing
    models
models of nursing, *see* care models; nursing
    models
moist (crackles), BPAF definition, before
    refinement 112
Moller-Murphy   Symptom   Management
    Assessment Tool 6–7, 8
mood change, BPAF definition, after refine-
    ment 133

mouth, BPAF definitions
  coated mouth
    before refinement 114
    after refinement 127
  dry mouth
    before refinement 114
    after refinement 127
Mucositis Grading Scale, WHO 17
multitrait-multimethod matrix method 16
Murphy Wellness Model 8
muscular pain, BPAF definition, after refinement 136

nausea, BPAF definition
  before refinement 114
  after refinement 128
neonates, sepsis in, assessment tool 7, 9
neurological system
  abnormal physiological signs and symptoms, literature review 99–102
  see also central nervous system
NLIU, see nursing-led inpatient unit
nurse-patient relationship, assessment and 2
nursing assessment, see assessment
nursing diagnosis, general assessment guide 7
nursing-led inpatient unit (NLIU)
  background xv–xvi
  description 19–20
  patient outcomes 26
  Physical Assessment Framework
    first version 93–4
    second version 38, 91–2
nursing models 3–4
  definition 3
  Orem's self-care nursing model 4
  see also care models
nursing process 1, 3

odour, see under urine
oedema, see pitting oedema
Oral Assessment Guide (OAG) 17
Orem's self-care nursing model 4
oxygenation section, of the BPAF 23

pain, see abdominal pain; calf pain; chest pain; joint pain; micturition; muscular pain
Pain Flow Sheet (PFS), construct validity 17
pale, BPAF definition

before refinement 116
  after refinement 125
paraesthesiae, BPAF definition, after refinement 133
parallel forms reliability testing 11
patient assessment, see assessment
phlegm, see sputum
physical assessment 87–90
  aims 87
  cardiovascular system 88
  carrying out 87–90
  central nervous system 90
  gastrointestinal system 89
  general points 90
  genitourinary system 89
  guidelines 87
  literature review 28
  respiratory system 88–9
  see also assessment
pitting oedema, BPAF definition
  before refinement 113
  after refinement 125
pleural rub, BPAF definition, after refinement 122
poor appetite, BPAF definition
  before refinement 114
  after refinement 127
predictive validity 14–15
pressure areas, reddening of, BPAF definition
  before refinement 116
  after refinement 137
problem identification, v. assessment 2
pulse rate
  BPAF definitions, before refinement 31, 112–13
  see also heart rate
purulent wound, BPAF definition
  before refinement 116
  after refinement 137

rash, BPAF definition, after refinement 136
reddening of pressure areas, BPAF definition
  before refinement 116
  after refinement 137
reduced tissue turgor, BPAF definition
  before refinement 113
  after refinement 127
reliability, of assessment tools 10–13
  as equivalence 11–12

inter-rater reliability 11–12
   as internal consistency 12–13
   parallel forms reliability testing 11
   as stability 10–11
   test-retest reliability 10–11
reliability of the BPAF, evaluation study
      39–63
   aims and objectives 40
   analysis
      of nominal data 44–5
      of ratio data 46–7
   approach taken 39–40
   data analysis techniques 44–7
   data collection preparation 42–3
   data collection process 43–4
      on the acute wards 43–4
      on the NLIU 43
   discussion 73–8
      nominal data 73–4
      nominal data, factors affecting 74–5
      ratio data 75–6
      ratio data, factors affecting 76–8
   ethical issues 41
   findings 47–62
   inter-rater agreement 46
   inter-rater reliability
      of BPAF as a whole 59–62, 78
      experienced assessors on acute wards
         54–5
      experienced v. novice assessor 55–9
      independent assessors on NLIU 48–50
      stability over time 43, 50–4
      summary 62–3
   method of investigation 40–3
   pilot work 42
   sample 40–1
   site 41
respiration
   abnormalities of, BPAF definitions
      before refinement 112
      after refinement 120–1
   added sounds, BPAF definition, after
      refinement 122
respiration section (original), of the BPAF 25
respiratory rate
   affecting inter-rater reliability 78
   BPAF definitions
      before refinement 112
      after refinement 120

respiratory system
   abnormal signs and symptoms, literature
      review 29–30
   physical assessment 88–9
Rogers' Science of Unitary Beings 7, 8

Science of Unitary Beings 7, 8
self-care nursing model 4
sepsis in neonates, assessment tool 7, 9
skin, BPAF definitions
   clammy skin, after refinement 126–7
   colour
      before refinement 116
      after refinement 125
   cool skin
      before refinement 115
      after refinement 126–7
   hot skin
      before refinement 115
      after refinement 126
   ulceration/damage
      before refinement 116
      after refinement 137
slurred speech, BPAF definition
   before refinement 117
   after refinement 133–4
spasticity, BPAF definition, before refine-
      ment 116–17
special diet feeding, BPAF definition
   before refinement 114
   after refinement 129
speech, defective, BPAF definitions
   before refinement 117
   after refinement 133–4
split-half technique 13
sputum, BPAF definition
   before refinement 37, 112
   after refinement 37, 121
stability
   of assessment tools 10–11
   medical stability xv, 20
stiffness, BPAF definition, after refinement
      135–6
stomatitis, chemotherapy-induced, staging
      system 6
stool, BPAF definitions
   constipated stool, before refinement 115
   hard/dry stool, after refinement 129
   loose stool

before refinement 115
    after refinement 129–30
stridor, BPAF definition, after refinement
    122
swelling, BPAF definitions
    calf
        before refinement 113
        after refinement 124
    joints/tissue, after refinement 136

tachycardia 123
temperature, see body temperature
test-retest reliability, of assessment tools
    10–11
tingling, BPAF definition, before refinement
    117
tissue swelling, BPAF definition, after refine-
    ment 136
tissue turgor, reduced, BPAF definition
    before refinement 113
    after refinement 127
turgor, see reduced tissue turgor

ulceration, BPAF definitions, see under skin
urgency, BPAF definition, after refinement
    131
urinary incontinence, BPAF definition
    before refinement 115
    after refinement 132
urinary symptoms, assessment tool 7
urine
    concentrated, BPAF definition
        before refinement 114
        after refinement 131
    odour, BPAF definition
        before refinement 114
        after refinement 131
utilization of the BPAF, evaluation study
    26–8

discussion 79–81
    action on detection of new abnor-
        mality 80–1
    frequency of completion 79–80
method 26–7
results 27–8

validity, of assessment tools 13–17
    concurrent validity 14
    construct validity 15–17
    content validity 14
    convergent validity 16, 17
    criterion-related validity 14–15
    definition 13
    divergent validity 17
    face validity 14
    predictive validity 14–15
validity of the BPAF, evaluation study, see
    content validity of the BPAF
visual disturbance, BPAF definition
    before refinement 117
    after refinement 132
vomiting, BPAF definition, after refinement
    128

weekly weight, BPAF definition
    before refinement 114
    after refinement 127
weight, see weekly weight
Wellness Model 8
Western Consortium for Cancer Nursing
    Research (WCCNR) 6, 9, 17
wheeze, BPAF definition
    before refinement 112
    after refinement 122
wound, purulent, BPAF definition
    before refinement 116
    after refinement 137